MY BODY AFTER PREGNANCY

WHAT YOUR FRIENDS DON'T TELL YOU

J. M. STAUFFER
B. L. HARRINGTON, B.S.N., R.N.

DEDICATION

To my late, loving mother. I'm sorry for being such a snotty teenager. I now understand what you went through after five kids of your own. I wish I could apologize to you in person. I love you.

To my wonderful mother-in-law. Thanks for having six amazing children. Thanks for having one in particular. Without him, I wouldn't have experienced the joy of having my own children.

ACKNOWLEDGMENT

Thank you to my good friend Trisha Carnahan, who lit a fire under me. You are the reason I wrote this book. You guided me through my first pregnancy. You helped me prepare for my baby's arrival, planned my baby shower, and laughed with me through the trials and tribulations of childbirth. You were my friend to call whenever I thought something was going wrong. You're funny, clever, and always someone I can rely upon.

Thank you to my sister-in-law, Kathy DeWolf, who shared her childbirth experiences. You encouraged me to finish the book and to share my stories in the hopes of helping other mothers. You gave me honest feedback, and throughout the process, you made me feel "normal." You are kind, smart, and patient. I hope my girls grow up and become amazing women just like you.

Thanks to my friends and family, especially my children, who let Mommy work on her computer. Thanks to my husband, who pushed me to write for at least an hour a day in between working and taking care of children.

Thanks to Brenda Harrington, who helped write and edit the book. You gave me funny verbiage and provided me with scientific information. You encouraged me from the start. You always see the glass half full. You're funny, hip, and can light up a room with your presence. I enjoy working with you. Let's get going on book number two in the series.

Thank you to Abby Wilson and Simone Martinez. My children adore you. You gave me and my husband precious time together. You allowed us to escape for date night and connect with each other, alone, without kids!

Thanks to Mike Murphy and the tennis pros at Carriage: Scott, Lexi, Jason, and Alex, for getting my butt moving again!

A big thanks to Suzanne Raney, who patiently helped edit and format the book. You were a driving force in putting the final piece of the puzzle in place!

As a first-time self-publisher, the journey can be frustrating, especially the road to the printing process. So, a huge thank you to Reedsy, and in particular, Elizabeth Ridley and Veronica Scott."

And lastly, thanks to Cornelia Sjoblom and her amazing cousin, Jim Sjoprank. Your skill, vision and unyielding talent in production and editing helped produce funny and kitschy videos. Catch them on YouTube.

CONTENTS

PREFACE

Congratulations, you just had a baby!

Your body has been on an incredible journey, and it has paid a hefty toll along the way.

For the last nine months, it has been subjected to fluctuating hormones, stretched skin, painful ligaments, tender breasts, a leaking bladder, prodded and relocated organs, breathing difficulties, indigestion, fatigue, swollen feet, and weight gain. Let's also not forget that for the last six weeks, your body's been running on E for Empty in the sleep department. It may have taken all the mental and physical energy you could muster to perform a simple task, like "rolling" out of bed in the morning. Yes, E for Exhausted, yet at the same time, Excited. Like the majority of first-time mothers, you're probably so relieved the "Big Day" has arrived—not only to receive your precious bundle of joy but also to reclaim your body and to get back to normal finally. Normal? Yeah, right!

If you're anything like me, you're thinking, "It'll only be a few weeks, or at most a few months, before my body's back to normal, and I'm sliding into my trusty, comfortable pair of jeans." After all, Heidi Klum had her fantastic, sexy bod back four weeks after having her baby. Madonna looked better than ever after having her babies, and, although it took Kate Hudson four months to look fabulous, she'd put on a whopping sixty pounds during one of her pregnancies. It all sounds easy enough, right?

Hindsight is 20/20, and, unfortunately, the EASY return to "normal" I expected once my baby arrived didn't materialize. Throughout my first pregnancy, I thought nothing of shoveling an extra piece of pie into my mouth, along with an extra scoop or two of ice cream. Sure, super-size my French fries to go along with my double cheeseburger. Why not? I ate what I wanted, when I wanted. I ate because I felt miserable during the last few weeks of my pregnancy, and food made me happy. For the first time in my life I had an excuse to overindulge. After all, I was eating for two. And eating was one of the few comforts I had left.

I couldn't relax at the end of the day with my familiar glass of wine because I couldn't drink alcohol. And oh, how I wanted comfort. I ached in areas of my body I couldn't scratch without assistance. I couldn't bend over far enough to put on or take off my shoes. I cut myself shaving because I couldn't see what I was shaving. It was hard work even to get in and out of the car. Food made me feel good. All I could think about was food. "Yeah," I thought, "I can lose the weight and get my body back after I have the baby. It'll be a piece of cake."

Unless you have a private chef and a personal trainer

spending three to four hours a day yelling at you to work those abs and tighten those buns, the road back to normal is a long one. The reality is that "nine months on, nine months off" is only accurate if you work extremely hard. After all, there's nothing natural about losing baby weight quickly. And there's a lot working against it. You still ache after having the baby; your appetite increases while you're breastfeeding; you're sleep-deprived, which is a big kick in the pants. Not sleeping means your brain produces less leptin, the hormone that turns on your food willpower switch, and without that, you want to overeat and overeat again. Did someone say, "cheese-burger" or "pie?" Did I mention that eating made me feel good? Sex was off the table for six weeks after having the baby, but carbs could give me the same euphoric experience. When I started to breastfeed, my body craved chocolate, pasta and fruit pie. A healthy salad didn't make it back on my list of deli-cious and comforting treats for months after giving birth.

This book is here to let you in on a few secrets about what to expect from your body after pregnancy. It took me eleven years to write, but over those years, I've come to understand my body's metamorphosis into, well, a "mom's" body. I've also identified the weird sensations and changes my body experi-enced along the way, and now understand that most were quite normal. Having the "baby blues," for example, is a real thing. Some women experience postpartum depression (PPD) or postpartum post-traumatic stress disorder (PTSD); it's much more than a weird feeling of sadness. It can be devastating. Then there are the bodily functions, or lack of, that go haywire postpartum. Nobody warns you, not your mom, not your sister (thanks, Sis), not your aunts, and indeed not your friends who, by the way, had the perfect pregnancy and are currently caring for the perfect baby. Not even my obstetrician let me in on what was about to go on with my body after pregnancy. When unfamiliar things started happening, I began to think I must be doing something wrong or that something must be wrong with me. The fear of the unknown only heightened my anxiety. I now understand that I wasn't alone. This book is here to prepare you for some of those surprising and strange bodily encounters that would have been reassuring to know about BEFORE I thought I was losing my ever-loving mind!

Maybe, like me, you don't realize what you're going through until you discover it's a real thing and, very likely, quite common. As a new mother, your body has suffered one of the most traumatic experiences a human body can encounter. Your body has spent nine months growing a whole new person inside of it, sharing and transferring nutrients, changing shape, stretching and expanding, and producing a plethora of hormones. But in a matter of hours, that life growing inside you is abruptly pulled out. Talk about life-changing!

You may feel like you're stumbling in the dark without a flashlight. Not anymore. This book, like Motel 6, will "Leave the Light on for You." I'll walk you through many of the changes your body may experience, from unexpected leakages to fits of uncontrollable tears.

This is not a medical book; instead, it is a personal compendium; an autobiographical journey peppered with insight from my good friend and nurse extraordinaire, Brenda Harrington, R.N., B.S.N. I want new mothers to know there's no such thing as an "easy" return to a pre-pregnancy body. Just like during pregnancy, we try whatever we can to get through each day as it comes.

I'm also here to let you know that there's no such thing as a "Super Mom." Look at yourself in the mirror every day and tell yourself, "I'm Super, and I'm a Mom!" Remember that most of what you're feeling and experiencing after pregnancy is normal—a new normal. And, just as every pregnancy can be different, your experience after pregnancy can differ from one birth to the next. So, ladies, if this isn't your first rodeo, or if you're giving birth for the very first time, read on; some things may surprise you!

SECTION ONE

CHAPTER 1:

THE BIG DAY

So, finally, labor and delivery are over. Given all goes well, your obstetrician, doula, or midwife has handed you a warm, tiny, reddish, brownish, or yellowish-looking thing for some valuable skin-to-skin time. You may be thinking the only thing you have to push from now on is a baby stroller. You have a newborn miracle in your arms. But don't worry if there isn't an instant connection like in the movies. You've just been through a stressful experience, and now you're expected to share this cinematic moment of instant mother-and-baby bonding. That certainly didn't happen to me. I had pushed so hard I felt like my head was going to pop off. Once my baby finally emerged, I felt seriously relieved I hadn't given myself an aneurysm. I was also incredibly drained. And hungry.

During delivery, my OB informed me I have a small pelvic opening. Could we not have discovered this minor detail before my eyes bugged out of my head, and I pooped all over the labor and delivery staff? (Yeah, that's a real thing, as we'll discuss later.) My baby's shoulders couldn't fit through my "small pelvic opening." Her head was small enough to slide through, but not the rest of her, so no matter how hard I pushed, she wasn't going to come into the world without a bit of intervention. I sensed the frustration of my doctor, who believed I didn't understand the word "push." After ten hours of labor, the situation became Code Red. The baby was in distress. Her heart rate plummeted. Fetal monitoring machines were going bonkers. My OB jumped into action, and the next thing I knew, I had several nurses sitting on my stomach. There was no time for an emergency C-section.

I knew I was in good hands because my OB was not only well seasoned in delivering little people, he also owned a cattle ranch and had plenty of experience reaching inside cows to bring their babies into the world safely. I grew up watching the veterinarian comedy series called *All Creatures Great and Small*, and each episode invariably opened with James Herriot's arm buried shoulder-deep in a cow's rear end. The outcome was usually the delivery of a healthy calf, so I wasn't overly concerned at this point. With that said, my OB thrust his hand into my vagina and broke my baby's left clavicle. After a quick tug, Voila! My beautiful baby girl was born.

A coterie of OB nurses cleaned her, weighed, and measured her. One of the nurses calculated her Apgar score and gave her a nine out of ten. Not bad for a baby who caused the monitoring machines to ring off the hook during labor. My doctor evaluated her clavicle and bandaged her shoulder. Then she was swaddled snuggly in a warm blanket and placed in my arms. A nurse instructed me to loosen or take off my gown and place my baby on my naked chest for some crucial skin-to-skin time. I later discovered that the first hour or so after birth is known as the "miracle hour," the "golden hour," or "sacred time." It's a time for momma and baby to feel each other's bare skin and listen to the rhythm of each other's heartbeat; an uninterrupted time that, according to studies, promotes newborn and maternal attachment, reduces stress, and helps a newborn transition into postnatal life. There's a great article on the National Institute of Health's website that details the benefits of skin-to-skin time, *Healthy Birth Practices #6 Keep Mother And Baby Together.*

As my baby lay comfortably on my chest, I kept thinking my OB was spending an excessive amount of time down there, fiddling. My feet were still in the stirrups. What was he doing? "I'm stitching you up," he chirped. He was surgically repairing the incision he'd made from my vagina to my anus. So, not only had he broken my baby's clavicle, but he'd also given me an episiotomy. OUCHY. I was feeling shocked, anxious, and exhausted. Thank goodness I was still pharmaceutically enhanced and under the influence of an epidural. The pain hadn't set in yet.

My small pelvic opening had caused my baby's face to bruise as I pushed her slowly through. She also had a very pronounced cone-shaped head. It's impressive how a baby's head can change shape and how the vaginal muscles stretch to accommodate childbirth, like a mouse fitting through a crack in a wall. Yet, despite what appeared to me as a traumatic birth, the medical staff assured me my baby was healthy, that her clavicle would heal quickly, and that she'd never know she suffered a broken bone.

After the realization that my baby was okay, my brain began to fantasize about big, juicy cheeseburgers. I imagined myself wolfing one down (extra mayo, ketchup, mustard, onions, and pickles) with a side of French fries (super-sized) and chasing it with an icy-cold drink and a long nap. It sounded blissful, and, as it turned out, only a brief fantasy. Now that my baby was no longer in my womb, the focus was no longer on me. I wasn't the center of attention anymore. I became just an item on a list of necessities a baby needs to flourish. Granted, I'm probably number one on the list, just above "diaper" and "warm blanket." I soon realized I had essentially become a food source for my baby. Everything happened so fast. The miracle hour had come to an end, my imaginary cheeseburger disappeared, and the next thing I knew, I had a nurse hovering by my bedside. I felt tugging, groping, squeezing. My breasts were no longer my own. They were no longer private property. Standing over me was a lactation specialist instructing me on how to get the baby to latch on. The baby needed feeding. NOW! Breastfeeding, by the way, is a learned skill. In my case, it certainly didn't come naturally. I'm not a mother goat with huge udders and four-inch long, drooping teats, as we'll discuss in a later chapter.

I talked to my sister-in-law about how tired and hungry I was after giving birth. She told me she felt the same way after her scheduled C-section. She hadn't eaten anything since bedtime the night before, and by five p.m. the following day, she was starving. The nursing staff wouldn't let her eat anything after delivery, not until she'd released either a fart or a bowel movement. But her cousin had brought her homemade peanut butter cookies, her favorite. She furtively scarfed down a dozen, and when the nurses discovered her secret, they threatened her with an enema. They were so irritated with her. She hadn't paid any attention to their warning, "NO SOLID FOOD IMMEDIATELY AFTER SURGERY!" They tried hard to give her a suppository, but her hemorrhoids were so swollen, there was no way on earth she would let anything penetrate her sore bum. And so she waited to cut the cheese.

Anytime we have abdominal surgery, our gut stops working as it should. It slows down or shuts down completely. Passing gas or pooping tells the nursing staff that your gastro-intestinal tract is waking up and starting to work normally again. Signs that it may be struggling to make a comeback include nausea, bloating, and abdominal pain. Although, how can you tell bloating from pregnancy tummy and abdominal pain from hunger pain, incision pain, or harmful gas pain? It all hurts down there![1]

If you're lucky, or you know what's good for you, you left your family and friends at home. However, chances are you have a slew of well-wishers pacing the floor of the hospital waiting room, counting the hours until they see you and—their primary motivation—meet your new baby. It's not all about you anymore. But if I were you, try to keep these cheer-leaders at bay for as long as you can. Instead, get some sleep. It would help if you had it. My advice is to get as much sleep

---

1   Check out the website *livescience.com, Why You Should Chew Gum Until You Fart After a C-section.* It references a study published online in the *Journal of Maternal-Fetal Neonatal Medicine* May 14th, 2017, suggesting that chewing gum after a C-section can jumpstart the gut into producing a fart sooner than women who didn't chew gum after surgery. Good to know. After delivering my second baby via C-section, I was lucky enough to fart shortly after delivery, which meant I could move on to hospital food, Jell-O, and liquid bullion (not a juicy cheeseburger, I seem always to crave). However, I did make sure I had a healthy supply of gum and stool softeners; there was no way I was going to allow my bum to cry, "Uncle," and submit to a suppository.

in the hospital as you possibly can. Think about it; the cost of my two-day hospital stay for vaginal delivery was around $14,000 after my insurance company negotiated discounts, and it would have cost more for a C-section delivery. For less than that, I could take my new family of three on a one-week vacation, flying first-class, to a Caribbean island and stay in a luxury villa complete with a chef, nanny, driver, butler, and magic clothes hamper. Instead, take advantage of your two days in a hospital bed! Enjoy the help you're given. You're worth it.

For a mere two days, I had nurses circling me, eager to show me how to change a diaper or swaddle my baby with a small blanket. These people are professionals who take care of babies every day. Unfortunately, my friend, you have quickly fallen from a pedestal and have now become sloppy seconds. So make sure you take care of yourself. Let the nurses take care of the baby while you SLEEP, SLEEP, SLEEP. And don't be afraid to ask for a sleep aid if you're in pain.

The second time around, I wised up and put my trust in the maternity nurses. I rented a hospital breast pump for twenty-five dollars a day. As soon as one of the nurses delivered the equipment to my room, I pumped enough colostrum to cover the first night's feeding. That evening, I asked the night nurses to take my baby to the nursery. As they turned their backs to head down the corridor, I downed a heavenly sleeping pill and fell into a deep sleep.

Meanwhile, the night nurses kept my baby safe and healthy as they fed her from a tiny pipet. They filled the pipet with the colostrum I'd pumped. The maternity staff knew what to do. I can't emphasize enough how important it is to have a good night's sleep, especially after all you've been through. Remember that we're only on day one, and you won't be able to take the maternity nurses with you when you go home. You'll no longer have professionals popping in and out of your room taking the utmost care of your baby. But don't worry, you'll maybe be able to get a good night's sleep again in, oh, about eighteen years!

SECTION TWO

CHAPTER 2:

THE "POOP SLIDE"

News alert, most women poop a little during childbirth. Your excellent medical staff effortlessly slide the poop away, clean it up, give you a quick wipe, and you're none the wiser. Farting and pooping are good signs during labor and delivery because it means that the baby is right on track and you're pushing correctly! Pooping is just a natural part of an incredible chain of events that helps the baby move through the birth canal and into our world. I don't precisely remember pooping, but I remember hearing the farts rip. Even though I had an epidural during my first labor and delivery, I could still feel pressure down below. I felt no pain from the waist down, thank goodness, but I could feel the pressure of pushing the baby. Something else I could feel was the sensation of my butt cheeks flapping. Undoubtedly, while I was cutting the cheese, I was sneaking out plenty of loose number twos, but if indeed I had pooped, my nurses were so adept at sliding the poop away that I was totally clueless. My husband was kind enough to tell me afterward that he recalled nothing except for our daughter coming into the world and recording her first cries on his cell phone. He was watching the birth through a full-length mirror my OB had placed at the end of the hospital bed. I guess all eyes were on the magic of the baby crowning.

The chain of events that causes us to poop is essential for delivering babies. It includes the release of prostaglandins in the uterus, which causes the uterus to contract, like when we have a period. The contractions cause the baby to move out of the womb and into the birth canal. As the baby gets lower in the birth canal, the pressure of the baby's head presses on receptors in the colon that tell the brain we need to poop. Also, pressure on the cervix gives us the urge to push. We're using the same muscles to push out the baby as we use to poop. As we push, the anal sphincter relaxes, and we all know what happens next.

What's a little gas and a little poop when the result is bringing a brand-new human being into the world? Besides, you're pushing out more than a baby, poop, and gas; there's the mucous plug, the bloody show, amniotic fluid, and some-times even the baby's pee and poop. How can the average lay-person tell what's what? So stay calm, push, and let it go.

CHAPTER 3:

THE "SUBWAY SANDWICH"

That's right. As soon as you leave the delivery room and sit comfortably in your hospital bed, you'll have a nurse come to your maternity floor to teach you how to build what my girlfriend and I affectionately call the "Subway Sandwich." Only, this isn't a tasty snack with lettuce, tomato, and pickles. It's a sandwich for your underwear. Yes, your underwear. This conversation is routine for the professionals, and they talk fast, so listen closely and pay attention to their demonstration. I was a little bewildered by the idea of what I had to strap into my panties; my hospital-issued, disposable, oh-so-sexy granny panties.

So, here's the drill. First, there's the most oversized panty pad you've ever seen in your life. I should rephrase that; the most oversized "sanitary napkin," because it looks like it came from the Dark Ages. The only thing this napkin is missing is the "belt." Your maternity nurse may be showing you the Super Overnight Pad. This one only measures twelve-and-a-half inches long by three inches wide. Or, she may be showing you the Queen Sanitary Napkin that measures a whopping fifteen-and-a-half inches long, basically from the top of the pubic hair to the end of the butt crack. The sanitary napkin reminds me of the filling used to make the "Subway Footlong Sandwich." It's like a wad of turkey, or a chicken cutlet. You'll have to wear this regardless of having a vaginal or cesarean birth. Your uterus will continue to discharge the remaining contents and lining over the next six weeks. Initially, it's bright red. And it's heavy, like a very heavy period. Hence the massive pad.

Next comes the ice pack, and it can come in several different forms depending on where you deliver. I was given a newborn diaper as an ice pack, one that had been soaked in water and thrown in a freezer until it was frozen solid. It was a Pampers diaper, I think. One of my friends who delivered in a different hospital received a genuine ice pack. It measured three inches wide and ten inches long. The icepack is what she used to sit on top of her disposable panties. It reminds me so much of the twelve inch loaf of bread, the base of the sub sandwich. So you figure the sandwich is approaching two inches high at this point.

Next, the witch hazel pads are laid on top to calm the badly swollen, bruised, stretched, and/or sliced perineum. Witch hazel rounds look so much like slices of delicious provolone cheese when you're feeling hungry, tired, and still a little groggy from an epidural. If your nurse is feeling generous, they may indulge and grant you extra rounds of cheese.

The final ingredient is the mayonnaise slather on top—a very-much-appreciated squeeze of pain-numbing Lidocaine cream or Dibucaine ointment. Please may I have some more?

And there you have it; you just received the recipe for creating the "Subway Sandwich!" You'll soon become proficient at making this yourself because every time you use the restroom, you'll discard the wet, bloody sandwich from your underwear and make up a fresh sub to last until your next visit to the bathroom.

If your doctor needed to perform an episiotomy, chances are you have stitches down there. Going to the bathroom will be painful. You'll benefit from taking a bidet-in-a-bottle with you every time you need to go. The bidet-in-a-bottle is an eight-ounce squeeze bottle filled with warm water, like the mustard or ketchup bottle you'll find at your local diner. You'll use it to shoot warm water around the area while you pee. It sounds weird but trust me, it helps big time. Every time I peed, it felt like shards of glass rubbing against my nether region. The warm water lessened the pain and helped clean the area simultaneously, like a very gentle bidet.

Having a baby totally takes the "rest" out of the restroom. Going to the bathroom is an ordeal. The crazy thing is, a few weeks after giving birth, the ordeal becomes less memorable. Nature has a beautiful way of muting bothersome memories of childbirth. Our mind/body experience doesn't always commit the pain and suffering to memory. After all, if these memories stayed with us, our newborns wouldn't have any brothers or sisters. You and I wouldn't have any brothers or sisters. We wouldn't have any aunts and uncles. Women would have to be crazy to go through this again. And yet we do. Fuzzy memory is the process of situational memory loss, and it comes in handy during traumatic events. Amnesia can be bliss.

CHAPTER 4:

GOING HOME—YIKES!

You may feel very apprehensive about going home and taking care of your little one(s) for the first time. I was petrified. I enjoyed my stay in the hospital, except for the pain and the exceptionally bland hospital food. I learned so much from my maternity nurses, OBs, and pediatricians, who continually popped in and out of my room.

I especially dreaded leaving the maternity ward and going home after my first baby because I knew I'd be on my own, for the first time, flying solo as a new mom. I didn't want my stay to end. I felt safe in my hospital bed with experts around me, waiting on me. I became pretty anxious when a nurse hurried into my room one afternoon and abruptly told me to get dressed, collect my belongings, and leave. My two-and-a-half-day stay (allowable by the insurance company for vaginal birth) had come to an end. I suddenly felt like a whore who'd done the dirty and was ordered to pick up her panties and leave hastily. No snuggling, no pleasantries, simply a door slam and a, "Get Outta Here!"

Minutes later, a second nurse entered the room and examined the car seat we'd brought along to the hospital. She checked to make sure it was safe and that it hadn't expired. Well, I never. Until that moment, I had no idea a car seat had an expiration date stamped on the bottom.

Next, in rolled a wheelchair. Wait. What? They had this exit strategy thing down to a science, and they were double-teaming. A nurse pointed and ordered me to sit. Begrudgingly, I complied. One nurse demonstrated how to strap the baby securely into the car seat while my husband and I stared like two deer in the headlights. After sitting the car seat on my lap, off we went. She wheeled me out of the maternity ward, passed the cafeteria (cheeseburger, anyone?), and outside to the nearest hospital curb.

And that's when I panicked. My husband and I had only taken care of ourselves our whole lives. We were both the youngest of multiple siblings; we're the babies. Now we had to take care of someone else completely, a whole other person, handle their every need? We had to become responsible parents, with no handbook? We felt kicked to the curb, alone, and in a stressful situation for first-time moms and dads.

Trying to plan, I had arranged for my husband's parents to come and stay with us once the baby was born. I felt better knowing they'd be able to calm my fears and lend experienced helping hands. After all, they had already gone through this six times—my husband has five siblings. I figured they'd have all the answers to my questions, from explaining the strange twinges I was feeling here and there to the unfamiliar bodily fluids my body was presenting. My mother-in-law, I thought, would be able to explain what was happening to me; she would be able to help and reassure me. Or maybe not. Remember nature's way of helping us forget the rigors of childbirth? Yeah, you guessed correctly, my in-laws had forgotten most of the nitty-gritty details. Besides, Grandma hadn't given birth in more than forty years, back during the days when childbirth included a week-long hospital stay when nurses took care of the newborns and provided lots of education and pearls of wisdom. Help was available to bathe the baby and take care of the fluids spewing from a new mom's undercarriage. Today, all we get is a fleeting one-to-two-day stay and a pamphlet (as if we have time to read it) with a list of dos and don'ts. On the plus side, we have pain medicines now, episiotomies aren't routine anymore, time with our babies isn't rationed or scheduled, and new mothers aren't treated like they have an illness.

Since the dawn of the internet, we're lucky to have a plethora of information available at our fingertips; however, too much information can be dangerous. There's the added stress of googling diseases and ailments and subsequently becoming a hypochondriac with a newborn baby. It can make your head spin. I was so afraid of Sudden Infant Death Syndrome (SIDS) or falling asleep during breastfeeding and dropping my baby on the floor. How would I know if something was really wrong with my baby? What if she had a heart defect? How would I know? Then there are the obvious questions like, how will I know when to feed my baby? Remind me how to change a diaper again? How do I swaddle? What do I do to stop the crying? The incessant crying! I soon discovered that newborn babies eat when they're hungry, sleep when they're tired, and the more love and attention they receive, the better.

Perhaps you have invited your parents or your in-laws to come and stay. In retrospect, I realized the invitation should have waited a week or two. Here's why: I needed time to bond, not only with my new baby but with my husband, together as new parents. I needed my husband to hold me and comfort me during bouts of crying for no apparent reason. I needed time to figure out my new post-pregnancy body. I needed time to become more mobile, to at least be able to go to the bathroom without screaming in pain, and I needed time to adjust and absorb all the advice I was about to receive.

I felt as though the timing of overnight guests could have

been much better. My husband spent more time feeding and entertaining his parents than he did taking care of me. I know that our company wanted to help, but mostly they wanted to hold the baby. All my body wanted to do during my baby's first week of life was to protect her at all costs and safeguard her single-handedly. I rejected the hands that so earnestly wanted to help. I was incredibly stingy and possessive with my newborn. I wanted to hold her and never let go. I didn't want anyone else to get in on the act, not even my husband. She was mine, and she belonged to me. I'd worked hard to bring her into this world, and in my mind, I was the only person who could adequately take care of her. I behaved like a spoiled child, not wanting to share her new toy. It was a solid week or two before I calmed down and happily handed her over. I shared her with friends and family, but only if I was close by, and only if they washed their hands first or I sprayed the crap out of them with hand sanitizer (the Luvs diaper commercials make much more sense after having a baby).

Besides, there's a magical thing that happens after you come home from the hospital. For the first week or two, your body runs on a heavenly dose of adrenaline. For me, it was a time when sleep deprivation wasn't in my vocabulary. It seemed effortless to get up two or three times a night to feed the baby and still have plenty of energy to sail through the next day.

This high-octane energy level lasted only a short time, however. Soon enough, exhaustion and reality set in. Coincidentally, or not, my baby began to sleep less and less during the day. She became more alert, she wanted to socialize, and more and more, she wanted the comfort of being held. She would scream when I wasn't paying her enough attention. And that's when I truly understood the meaning of E for Empty. I felt exhaustion like I'd never felt before. Pregnancy Empty paled in comparison. If I was lucky enough to enjoy a mere four hours of sleep, it seemed like I'd embarked on a dream vacation.

My sister-in-law felt the same way about her daughter after her delivery. Her baby became the most important thing in her universe. She thought no one could love her child as much as she did. No one could protect her or keep her safe as well as she could. Her husband, the baby-daddy, shouldn't even think about taking care of her; what can he offer? She felt as though she was living on a full-on adrenaline cocktail. Her feelings were so intense that she couldn't sleep; she was too focused on making sure her baby was breathing while sleeping in her crib. She was obsessed with her baby's needs and that her baby was getting enough love, enough skin-on-skin time, enough milk, enough attention to grow. My craziness was similar. I slept on the floor next to my baby's bed for a few nights after returning home from the hospital to make sure she was breathing. With baby number two, I bought a bassinet that stayed next to my bedside. Protecting my babies became a fixation. Luckily, a week or two later, like the fog of a hangover, the adrenaline wore off, and all I wanted to do was sleep.

But by that point, paternity leave was over, my husband went back to work, my in-laws drove the three-hour trip home, and I was all alone to take care of my tiny infant. I was scared all over again and, I hate to admit, a little resentful.

A week or two postpartum is the ideal time for the parents or in-laws to come visit because not only do you long for sleep, you long for somebody to take the baby, even if it's for just an hour or so. I was so appreciative of any help I could get; I needed a break for simple pleasures, like showering in peace, brushing my teeth, washing my hair, or shaving my legs. You know, a basic hygiene routine. This was the time when I needed the love, reassurance, and support of my relatives. Please come back!?

CHAPTER 5

TUMMY ACHES AND PAINS

I'm sure you heard this a million times from your OB over the last nine months—our pregnant bodies have about fifty percent more blood volume than our pre-pregnancy bodies. You probably haven't heard that we don't lose all of this extra blood and uterus lining during delivery. No, no, postnatal bleeding can last for several weeks afterward. That's right; just when I thought the birthing gig was over, I discovered I had a six-week-long period to look forward to with a side order of stomach cramps. Don't be too hasty to trash those hospital-issued granny panties and monster "sanitary" napkins. You have only one option for the next few weeks, and that is to wear pads: doctor's orders, nothing in the vajayjay for six weeks, nothing from the twentieth century anyway, like tampons.[2]

---

2   Sidebar, Chella Quint (menstrual activist, performer, and #periodpositive founder) wrote an article published in The Independent in 2017 that railed on the pad and tampon industry. She has a valid point. The words "sanitary," "feminine," and "hygienic" are names that invoke shame and secrecy around having periods. She's pushing to rename these products "disposable menstrual products" instead. Companies imply their menstrual products are

Just an FYI, the term "hygiene" associated with menstrual pads developed around the turn of the twentieth century. It arose out of concern that the prevailing method used could harbor bacteria. Ladies at the time relied on reusable home-made cloths, and if they weren't thoroughly cleaned between each use, bacteria could grow. Check out a great article by Jennifer Kotler, Ph.D. published on helloclue.com entitled, *A Short History of Modern Menstrual Products.*

Like me, you may experience painful cramps, just like menstrual cramps. That's because the uterus continues to contract even after delivery. At first, it cramps to detach the placenta from the uterus wall; then, it contracts to heal itself after the placenta separates. It sounds weird, but when our body heals a cut on our skin, it produces blood clots to stop the bleeding. Our uterus acts differently. It doesn't heal ouch-ies with blood clots; instead, it contracts to "squeeze" the blood vessels shut. This way, there's no scarring left behind, like scars left behind on our skin from a cut. This method of

---

cleaner than women's bodies by using such terms, but disposable products aren't more sanitary, more feminine, or more hygienic than reusable products, and periods aren't any more unsanitary than other bodily functions. Chella points out that vaginas are actually self-cleaning, like ovens! Yep, I'd never thought of my vagina as a self-cleaning organ, but the low pH, abundance of healthy bacteria, and natural secretions help keep it clean. From now on, the term we'll use is disposable pads. Let's embrace our periods and be proud of the products we purchase from the confounded "Feminine Hygiene" aisle!

closing the placenta attachment site is "involution." A new embryo can't attach to scar tissue in the uterus. What a newly fertilized egg needs is thickly lined tissue that's rich in blood for it to burrow into, attach, and grow. Without the miracle of involution, we'd have no brothers or sisters, aunts or uncles.

I found that wearing a belly band helped. The idea of wearing a band after birth goes way back. Maybe even to the Dark Ages (along with the huge disposable pad complete with belt)! Back in the day, they were probably known as corsets or girdles. Today, we have a slew of names for them—postpartum belt, belly wrap, band, binder, belly-shrinker, and even the Kim Kardashian waist trainer. There are different-sized bands and different levels of compression depending on their purpose. Some are purely for aesthetics, cinching hard to suck in the extra pounds. But note that a hard cinch is not recommended for a postpartum belly. If you're thinking of buying a band, the type of band you choose also depends on whether you've had a vaginal birth or a C-section.

I grew up in England, where Jell-O is known as jelly (and what's known as "jelly" in the US is called "jam"). I remember watching jelly adverts on the telly (or TV commercials for Jell-O). The jingle was a catchy little number that chanted the words, "Jelly wobble on a plate!" And the visual was an enormous blob of Jell-O wiggling on a plate the size of a serving platter; an apt metaphor for my post-pregnancy stomach sans the belly band. Wearing the band not only made my belly look better, but it also felt better. Once I was up and about, I felt as though I had better posture and stability when lifting and carrying my baby. It helped calm my cramping, and after my second pregnancy, it helped protect my C-section stitches and incision.

I wore the belly band soon after delivery and kept it on for a few weeks afterward. I wore it night and day. I didn't shower much during the first few weeks, so I didn't have to take it off very often. My maternity nurses warned me not to tighten the Velcro straps too tightly because too much pressure can cause slow healing. When I asked if it would help me lose weight, they may have laughed a little. I guess the belly band allows the uterus to shrink more quickly; it's not a weight-loss device but more of a catalyst to help the uterus contract. Bummer. It can take weeks for the uterus to shrink, much to the dismay of one of my girlfriends who was expecting it to happen overnight. After leaving the hospital from delivering her first baby, she was so surprised her tummy still looked as if she was six months pregnant. Leaving the hospital after having a baby is nothing like leaving a wedding to change into a sexy honeymoon outfit. Word of advice, bring comfortable, generously sized clothes to the hospital for your departure.

One of the reasons our tummy looks round and squishy after delivery is because the uterus still cradles the leftovers from childbirth. The baby accounts for only a fraction of the additional weight we add during pregnancy. In my case, sixty-six pounds minus seven pounds eight ounces, leaving a whopping fifty-eight pounds eight ounces. I really didn't think about the math until after I had the baby.

Lochia is the official name given to postpartum bleeding, and it's your body's way of getting rid of all the junk left over from childbirth—whether you had a vaginal birth or a C-section. It's like having a very heavy period, only it's more than just blood. It's placenta tissue, mucus, small blood clots, and blood. It usually starts just hours after the baby is born and, in the beginning, it's bright red. By the end, it's typically whitish or yellow-white, so don't freak out! We're used to having periods that start a little brownish, then transition to red and taper to a darker red/brown. An abundance of white junk in my undies usually tells me I'm horny. Yellow usually means I peed myself or that I could have an infection of some sort. In the case of lochia, not so much. Being horny was the furthest thing from my mind; peeing myself, on the other hand, had become a problem. Postpartum urinary incontinence is a subject I'll explore in another chapter. Remember, no tampons until you get the green light from your physician at your six-week checkup; your only option is the big, old menstrual pad. A tampon would be worthless, anyway.

Some of the blood clots I passed scared me. They looked like chunks of raw liver. Whatever you do, please don't allow your pup to join you in the restroom; it'll go crazy with the musty smell of blood and the sight of what appears to be raw meat. My girlfriend told me she was surprised by the smell—stale and musty, and for the first few days, every time she stood up, she gushed. By the way, if you have excessive bleeding, you may be experiencing postpartum hemorrhaging. Some signs may be that you soak a thick panty pad in less than an hour, or you're passing large blood clots considerably larger than the size of a plum. You may or may not feel dizzy or even faint. One to ten percent of postpartum pregnancies can experience hemorrhaging, and it can start anywhere from birth to six weeks afterward. If this happens to you, call or see a doctor quickly. Or better yet, go to the ER. Get professional help. Hemorrhaging is no joke.

My maternity nurses also suggested I help the uterus along with daily massaging. I wondered where I would find the time to give myself a massage every day. One of my girlfriends sent her husband to the local pharmacy to pick up oxytocin (brand name Pitocin). Not to be confused with the pain killer OxyContin, oxytocin is a naturally occurring hormone that causes cervical dilation during labor and uterine contractions after labor. We release it naturally in response to nipple stimulation (from the baby rooting and feeding); it helps our milk "let-down" for breastfeeding. On a side note, it's also known as the "love hormone" and has a role in orgasm. Hmmm, nipple rubbing may have been the precursor to this situation I find myself in right now. But that's another story.

Remember to always get the okay from your OB or medical professional before buying any aids, bands, or supplements.

CHAPTER 6:

MY BEAUTIFUL BREASTS, WHAT HAPPENED?

After childbirth, you'll soon realize that your breasts have a purpose other than tantalizing your partner and looking spectacular in a push-up bra and tight t-shirt. They go through so many changes, beginning in early pregnancy. I first suspected I was pregnant because my boobs became extremely sensitive. My husband didn't believe me. He had to see three positive pregnancy stick tests, and even then, he thought the lines were so faint they didn't count. But I knew what my boobs were telling me. I enjoyed the larger size of my breasts during pregnancy, but not the additional soreness and tenderness. After my baby was born, I experienced more new and weird sensations to the point I seriously wondered if the "girls" would ever want to party again.

For a start, there's the uncomfortable feeling of breast engorgement; cracked, sore nipples; random nipple leakage; and the occasional infection with or without plugged milk ducts. As if we didn't have enough to deal with in other areas of our body—our body takes the discomfort level up a notch by adding breastfeeding to the list of painful distractions to getting our bodies back to normal. After breastfeeding comes breast ptosis or saggy tits...

Good breastfeeders always like to talk about how long they breastfed, like it's a symbol of their excellent mothering. Showoffs! And we're told ad nauseam that the earlier and longer a baby is breastfed, the better. As new mothers, our doctors, friends, frenemies, and baby development books remind us of the benefits of breastfeeding—from building a healthy immune system for our newborn to establishing long-term psychological benefits of bonding with our child. Both the American Academy of Pediatrics and the World Health Organization recommend breastfeeding exclusively for the first six months. The US Centers for Disease Control's website (cdc.gov/breastfeeding/data/facts.html) published data from the National Immunization Survey 2018-2019 that said an estimated eighty-four percent of mothers began breastfeeding their newborn babies in 2017. Six months later, twenty-five percent were still breastfeeding exclusively, and fifty-eight percent were breastfeeding and supplementing with formula or food. Overall, the survey states the majority of mothers don't breastfeed for as long as they initially intended. Why? BECAUSE IT'S NOT EASY! Why doesn't anyone ever tell us this? People may say there could be a couple of bumps along the way (excuse the pun), but then, in their next breath, they're talking about breastfeeding as a beautiful experience and how crucial it is for the baby. FYI, the CDC website lists a number of reasons why mothers don't breastfeed for as long as they set out to, and I'm quoting:

- Issues with lactation and latching

- Concerns about infant nutrition and weight

- Mother's concern about taking medications while breastfeeding

- Unsupportive work policies and lack of parental leave

- Cultural norms and lack of family support

- Unsupportive hospital practices and policies

I found breastfeeding frustrating and elusive, even though the key to making it work sounds quite simple—get the baby to latch on in the right spot. Breastfeeding is all about the areola. Never in my life have my areola had such a "special purpose," and never have they been so large or so dark. My once-perky nipples surrounded by pink, quarter-sized areolas transformed into flat nipples with milk-chocolate-colored, silver dollar-sized areolas that were peppered with white goosebumps. A new mom's areola can grow as large as four inches in diameter, which is about the size of my A cup during my twenties. They change to become more visible to the baby, like a bull's-eye, and our baby needs to get a big old mouthful of nipple and areola to breastfeed correctly—it's the secret to success. Although the white goosebumps looked a lot like juicy zits and were perfect for popping, I resisted the urge to squeeze them. They're actually Montgomery's tubercles, or sebaceous glands, that produce a germ-fighting, lubricating oil along with a slight odor to help the baby find the nipple.[3]

All I know is, mothers who are able to breastfeed well should carry a badge of honor to show for it. I didn't know what I was doing at first and ended up with all kinds of issues. Looking back, I needed expert advice. The instruction I received in the hospital after delivery wasn't very memorable, and at the time, I was tired and hungry. Shortly after the "miracle hour" ended, I had lactation specialists barge into my room and take control by shoving my breast into my baby's mouth. It was the kind of pulling and pushing reminiscent of a

---

3   The website *https://www.medela.com/breastfeeding/mumsjourney/* breast-changes-pregnancy-to-weaning quotes the following, "In fact, scientists believe the smell of this oil is similar to amniotic fluid and may help guide your newborn to your nipples after she's born."

mammogram. The specialists knew precisely what they were doing, but their groping and squeezing didn't give me the warm and fuzzies. I felt a little alarmed, confused, and violated. I guess their goal was to make sure my baby received my first milk, the precious colostrum, and with that goal in mind, they were successful. Perhaps I should have paid more attention and asked more questions, but exhaustion, hunger, and a terribly sore undercarriage took precedence.

I sucked at breastfeeding (no pun intended). After leaving the hospital, I discovered I couldn't provide enough milk to satisfy my newborn's needs. My baby was losing weight fast. When she was born, she weighed seven pounds, eight ounces, and when we left the hospital a couple of days later, she dropped to seven pounds, one ounce. No biggie, I thought, because it's normal for babies to lose a few ounces right away because they eliminate the amniotic fluid they ingested in the womb. My daughter, however, dropped an additional four ounces a couple of days later. She was continually crying, even though I was breastfeeding her every two or three hours. Finally, at two a.m., three days after we came home from the hospital, I called our pediatrician's office because I simply couldn't calm her down. He told me to buy formula and feed her a bottle ASAP. And just like that, I felt like a complete idiot. Why didn't I know to check the most common triggers of a baby crying? How did I not know she was most likely hungry, tired, or had a dirty diaper? I felt like an inadequate mother and questioned my ability to properly care for my infant when I couldn't even figure out something as simple as hunger.

I was in no state to drive, so my husband threw on his clothes and headed to the nearest twenty-four-hour pharmacy. It seemed like an easy task, "buy formula." Unfortunately, he was met with a slew of formula options and turned into a deer in the headlights. In addition to the host of different brands, there were different types, like infant formula, newborn formula, cow's milk allergy formula, gassy tummy formula, sensitive formula, Alimentum formula, soy milk formula, and Australian goat milk formula. The variety was endless. What to buy? He was the only person in the entire pharmacy other than the store clerk. He pulled a few containers from the shelf and headed for the checkout. He explained our situation and asked for help. The clerk recommended he buy a straightforward newborn formula, and he did just that. The magical powder was a life-saver! The container's instructions were simple to follow, and within minutes, my baby was sucking on a bottle like a baby goat at a petting zoo. At least with a bottle, I knew exactly how much milk my baby was consuming. For the next eight weeks, I pumped and pumped to stimulate the milk flow from my breasts while I continued to supplement with formula. I still struggled with breastfeeding weeks later and eventually gave up the idea altogether. I'm not sure what my problem was; were my breasts too engorged, causing flat nipples? A poor latch, football cleats for nipples before my milk came in, clogged milk ducts, low milk production? Word of advice: have a container of infant formula on hand and practice making up a bottle before delivering your baby. Don't think twice about calling a lactation specialist, either. Better safe than sorry.

BREAST ENGORGEMENT

Right after giving birth, our bodies produce our "first milk," known as colostrum. It's much thicker than our "mature" milk, which arrives a few days after delivery. We only make about one to four teaspoons of colostrum a day. It sounds like such a small amount of milk to feed a baby that weighs as much as a sack of potatoes, but believe it or not, it's just what our baby needs. A newborn baby's stomach is tiny— about the size of a small grape. You've probably heard that colostrum is so important because it provides our little one with many health benefits, including growth factors and antibodies for immune defense. It aids digestion by protecting against tummy upsets, and it works like a laxative to help get meconium, or baby poop, moving along. Maybe you haven't heard that colostrum supplements are available for grown-ups? I was surprised to learn that Amazon has a whole host of products costing twelve to seventy dollars a month. The pills, capsules, or powders are produced from the colostrum of goats and cows. They are touted as "superfood factors" with all kinds of benefits such as auto-immune defense, gastrointestinal help, support of lean muscle tissue, cell rebuilding, you name it. I have no idea if a goat's colostrum, dried and manufactured into pill form, is beneficial to an adult. However, I am convinced that a mother's colostrum given directly to a newborn is incredibly helpful for the baby. The website americanpregnancy.org has a great explanation of the benefits of colostrum. It's worth checking out *Colestorum—The Superfood For Your Newborn.*

"Mature" breast milk usually comes in about two to five days after the baby is born. At that point, breasts can become engorged. If that happens, they will feel hard. I knew as soon as it happened to me because my breasts felt full, firm, and very tender. My boobs were so tight I could bounce a quarter halfway across the room off either one. They were more sensitive than they were during pregnancy. Surprisingly, they even grew another couple of cup sizes; I was pushing an E cup from a B/C cup before pregnancy. Not only were my breasts filling up with milk, but they were "engorging" with increased blood flow to help prime the pump. They hurt. Here are a few things you may want to try to ease the discomfort of engorged breasts:

- Wear a supportive bra at all times. You may be able to pick up a cheap one at Walmart or Target that'll do the trick, but if not, invest in a decent one. You'll be wearing it 24/7. Remember, your breasts will be more massive than they were during pregnancy, so make sure you get the right size.

- Feed the baby every two to three hours to release the milk and ease the pain. Feeding regularly makes for a healthy feeding pattern for both your breasts and your baby—the old supply-and-demand trick. It's incredible how your breasts will learn to anticipate the next feeding.

- Massage the breast before feeding. It'll help prime the pump, and if you happen to have a clogged milk duct, which happens often, it'll help relieve it. Also, use a warm compress before feeding to get the stream flowing and a cold compress after feeding to ease the tenderness. A washcloth soaked with either warm or cold water will work well.

- Make sure you empty the breast during each feed—
  you'll hear this over and over again from lactation
  specialists, blogs, and books. Perhaps not from family
  and friends because they have fuzzy memories!

The baby gaining weight is the best way to measure if
breastfeeding is going well—it means your breasts are doing
their job, and the baby is getting enough milk. No need for a
midnight excursion to the pharmacy for formula.

It all sounds simple enough, right? It took a while for me
to figure it out. I believe my problem was that I became huge-
ly engorged, causing my nipples to flatten. My poor baby
didn't have anything to latch on to and ended up sucking away
on my skin. That, in turn, led to sore and cracked nipples, the
next topic of conversation.

SORE OR CRACKED NIPPLES

Cracked nipples are not something that develops overnight. Usually, you'll feel okay, for the first week or so of
breastfeeding, anyway. But when or if it happens, my God, it
hurts! After my deliveries, I took prescription pain killers because of episiotomy incision pain with my first delivery and
C-section incision pain with my second delivery. My pain tol-
erance with narcotics was higher than usual. Yet I cringed at
the thought of feeding my baby. For the first few seconds, as

my baby tried to latch, my nipples screeched in pain. It felt like someone was rubbing little pieces of glass in and around my nipple. Then, after a few seconds, it became bearable.

More often than not, my baby would hinge on the tip of my nipple and suck as hard as she could. I would physically flinch in pain, like a cow tangled in an electric fence trying to escape. I'd move her around, trying to hit the sweet spot so we'd both be doing better, but I just couldn't seem to get away with it. Even in the best of situations, it takes a week or so for nipples to toughen up to breastfeeding. It also takes about a week to figure out the baby's most comfortable positions to get a good latch. My advice is to persevere for as long as you can, and if you're able to get away with it, it's well worth the initial pain, clumsiness, and discomfort. You can find some great tips for getting through the soreness on the website *americanpregnancy.org*.

If you have to supplement your milk with formula, it's not the end of the world. I tried and tried to breastfeed and had every intention of breastfeeding exclusively for three months, but I had a hard time getting enough of my milk into the mouth of my baby. Maybe you find your milk doesn't come in, or you're hurting in too many other places to add breast pain and crusty nipples into the mix. Perhaps you choose not to breastfeed; whatever the reason, the most important thing is getting enough food for your baby. You don't owe anyone an explanation. The formulas on the market today are so good. They contain omega-3 fatty acids, including DHA (docosahexaenoic acid, which encourages healthy brain development), proteins, carbohydrates, iron, and other essential nutrients. Don't feel like your baby won't grow because you're not breastfeeding. Don't think that your baby's immune system will be compromised because you're feeding her formula. I know this is easier said than done, but try not to feel like you've failed as a mother, as I did. Don't let people shame you because you can't or won't breastfeed. At her nine-month checkup, my little one was in the fiftieth percentile for weight, head size, and height. My Little Miss Average had a diet consisting mainly of baby formula for the first few weeks of her life, and she didn't have a single drop of breast milk after about nine weeks. She's doing just fine, so move over, sore nipples!

I took to the internet and came across a few ideas to reduce the likelihood of further cracking or, even worse, turning cracked nipples into nasty breast infections. Some of the websites I visited were *verywellfamily.com*, *medela.us*, *americanpregnancy.org*, and *laleche.org.uk*. A quick acronym to remember, and not an official name by any means, is CLASS ACT:

- CALM. Take time to calm yourself and relax before feeding. Being anxious or tense can interfere with your milk letting down, which means your baby will be more demanding and suck even harder to get the milk they need; ouch!

- LATCH. First, the old adage, an ounce of prevention is worth a pound of cure. Ensure the baby is latched on properly, which means she's positioned correctly in your arms and clamped onto your areola, not your nipple—your nipple should be all the way to the back of your baby's mouth. Being in the wrong position while feeding is the number-one cause of sore nipples. I can attest!

- ADJUST POSITION. Try leaning back while you breastfeed. Sit on a comfortable nursing chair or prop yourself up on the couch with pillows. Bring the baby up to your nipple instead of hunching over and taking the nipple to your baby. Support her head with your arm or a nursing pillow.

- SOOTHE & MOISTURIZE. After feeding, massage your breast a little bit to squeeze out a few more drops of milk. Use the milk as a natural moisturizer to rub around your areola and nipple. Softer breasts help a good latch. Direct hit! Battleship! There are so many subtle (and some not so subtle) changes our body goes through—nuances of nature necessary to care for our newborn babies. Our breast milk also has natural antibacterial power. If you decide to use a store-bought nipple cream, make sure it's safe for the baby and doesn't contain alcohol.

- SUPPORT. Make sure you have the right-fitting bra to support those puppies and prevent chaffing.

- AIR-DRY. Air-dry your breasts before putting them away. This will prevent moisture from being trapped and irritating the skin. Change breast pads regularly and keep the site as dry as possible.

- CLEAN. Keep the area clean, using only warm water to wash with—no harsh chemicals, soaps, or exfoliating cleansers.

- TELL YOUR DOCTOR. See your doctor if the pain is excruciating, and consult a lactation specialist if you feel you need help.

If your nipples burn, you may have a yeast infection that will need an anti-fungal cream or an antibiotic to clear up. Other signs of a yeast infection are itchy, crusty, pink nipples. Very attractive! You may have caught it from your baby's mouth if she has a dose of thrush. Her tongue and the inside of her cheeks will have a thick, white, sometimes cottage cheesy-looking coating. Again, put in a call to your doctor's office to get some advice. The doctor may give you a prescription or tell you to pick up an over-the-counter cream.

My friend's nipples were so sore from breastfeeding, her doctor gave her a prescription cream. It was a compound mix of antibiotic, anti-fungal, and anti-inflammatory creams. She also called a lactation specialist, who basically told her that her nipples were too big for her baby's mouth. Rude! Flat nipples, football cleats for nipples, so many obstacles to a perfect latch!

LEAKY BREASTS AND IT'S NOT MILK...

Breast infections are no joke. It's a fairly common occurrence, and it can be excruciating. As if normal breastfeeding isn't painful enough! It feels like having your nipples twisted—a cruel and unusual punishment. *Webmd.com* says that breast infections are most likely to occur one to three months after delivery. Lactation mastitis, ironically pronounced *masty-tus* and not *mas-TIT-is*, is an infection caused by the bacteria staphylococcus or streptococcus.

Mastitis can be the result of milk backing up (milk stasis) and leaking into the breast tissue. It then becomes infected with bacteria growing in the swollen tissue. Milk stasis is the slowing or stoppage of the normal flow of milk. Clogged milk ducts are the most likely culprit, and clogged milk ducts can occur from a poor latch. Our breasts are producing milk, but our babies can't drink it fast enough, thus creating a backup in the boob.

Another cause could be pressure or trauma to the breast. Clothing that's too tight, an irritating underwire bra, a strap from a heavy diaper bag or a cinching seat belt, a hit, a kick, or a fall can all cause milk stasis. We can also pick up bacteria from our baby's mouth during breastfeeding. A cracked nipple is the perfect entry point into our system.

Lactation mastitis looks like a red or red-purple bruise. It can take over the whole breast, and it may feel hot, tender, and swollen. It may cause a fever, more clogged milk ducts, and of course, more pain. If the infection is detected early, your doctor can prescribe antibiotics that'll help to rid you of the condition. If not, it may turn into an abscess that will have to be lanced and drained, ouch! So, some tips to help prevent this ugly mess—keep your nipples clean and moisturized, wash them with a soft, clean, damp cloth after feeding, and don't use soap. There are plenty of nipple creams on the drugstore shelves, so pick one that is okay to use during breastfeeding. The goal is to keep the area supple to prevent the nipple from cracking. Also, bacteria thrive in stagnant milk, in or out of the breast. So, again, empty the breasts frequently. Pump if you have to and store any extra milk in the freezer. Don't wait until you have a festering mess on your hands!

Pregnancy and breastfeeding truly transform the "girls." And that's exactly what happened to me—from perky Mount Everests to a cross between saddlebags and south by southwest. Saggy tits—another souvenir of pregnancy. But having my kids is worth every pound of the floppy knockers I now sport.

CHAPTER 7:

YOUR REALLY, REALLY SENSITIVE SIDE

I have a friend who never used to cry in front of anyone. She was the Tin Man, with no emotion, no tears—not even during the movie *The Notebook*! Who doesn't cry during that movie? James Garner has been in love with his wife since they were teenagers, and when they become old, she has no clue who he is because she has dementia. They die in the same hospital, together, holding hands. For goodness' sake, that scene can make even the toughest of us cry. Since my friend's baby came along, she can't get through an ASPCA animal rescue TV commercial without reaching for a Kleenex. Sarah McLachlan, you're good! My friend's baby is now thirteen years old, and she still wells up at the drop of a hat. I'm the same way. On a scale of one to ten on the old Cry-Baby Richter scale, I was probably a two before pregnancy. Soon after the baby was born, I became a solid nine, maybe even a ten out of ten. Just call me the waterworks department. Don't be surprised if you feel like you're losing it after getting home from the hospital, especially when you see a diaper commercial on TV. Having a baby changes you.

Friends of another girlfriend visited her a few days after she arrived home from the hospital. They were excited to dote on her new little bundle of joy. Her husband welcomed them into their home and patiently entertained them while he waited for his wife and newborn baby to join them proudly. He waited and waited and finally went upstairs to see why they were taking so long. He was stunned to find his wife sitting on the floor in a corner of their bedroom, rocking back and forth, sobbing uncontrollably. Thinking something tragic had happened, he was ready to call 911. Fortunately, he soon realized mother and baby were safe. His wife was so upset because her clothes didn't fit her anymore. Her only options were her extra-large nighties or her end-stage maternity clothes. In her mind, she simply couldn't and wouldn't entertain guests wearing anything from her "size enormous and hideous" wardrobe. She broke down and refused to leave the bedroom, crying and screaming at her husband for not understanding the severity of her crisis. Her good friends eventually left that day without even a glimpse of her baby.

Hormonally, we're up and down. Compare it to a ride on the biggest, most badass roller coaster ride you can find at the amusement park. Only nothing is amusing about this ride. My emotional roller coaster sank to a new low after childbirth. Having a baby messed up my psyche. I used to be a pillar of mental strength, and then I became a pile of blubbering rubble.

I well up with tears every time I see or hear anything to do with children, good or bad. If I witness a kid falling and skinning a knee, I cry. If I watch a TV show and see a kid ride a bike without training wheels for the first time, I start bawling. If a stranger pays my child a compliment, a tear rolls down my cheek. I start sobbing at parent-teacher conferences when my daughter's teacher tells me my kid adds a ray of sunshine to her classroom every morning. I was the woman who didn't want anything to do with kids before having my own. I was the ice queen. Then I hit thirty-six, the clock started ticking, and my hormones took control. After that, all I wanted was to have a family. After having a baby, my emotions are at another level of whacky. I'm forever changed.

Think about what we're going through right now. We're experiencing a plethora of whammies. Not only are we battling hormonal fluctuations, but there's also the lasting exhaustion of childbirth, lack of sleep from feeding the baby every couple of hours, soreness, the discomfort of continually feeling wet down below, and the unfamiliarity of our new shape and size. There's massive anxiety about being responsible for a tiny human being who can't survive without us. What to do? How do women do this over and over again?

And then, all of a sudden, it all makes sense. We receive a coo or a smile from our little one. After we see and hold what we've created—what we grew inside of us—a brand-new person, life comes into perspective.

Thanks to estrogen and progesterone, we have a natural "upper" and a "downer" (*Women's Moods* by Dr. Deborah Sichel). Estrogen is the primary female sex hormone, and our ovaries produce most of it for us. Estrogen is a naturally occurring hormone in both men and women; the testes manufacture it in men. The adrenal glands and fat tissue also produce small amounts. Estrogen is a hormone with multiple functions as it helps keep our cholesterol in check, protects our bones, and affects our skin, heart, and brain (our mood). (*Hormone.org*) After childbirth, our hormones are completely out of sync, and it takes time for them to re-balance and stabilize. In the meantime, fluctuating estrogen levels may explain why we burst into tears for no apparent reason. It can explain our mood swings and feelings of irritability. Just know that no one really knows why we have the potential to go batty after childbirth, but low estrogen levels are thought to play a role. All this reminds me of an old joke, "How do you make a hor-mone? Don't pay her!"

Or, in the case of low estrogen levels, "Run for the hills!"

The "baby blues" is a normal state of affairs that affects up to eighty percent of new mothers. It's different from postpartum depression, which is a serious condition and may need professional intervention. The "blues" are usually mild and last anywhere from a few hours after childbirth to a week or two postpartum. It's not a psychiatric disorder. Feelings may include all or one of the following:

- Crying
- Feeling Down
- Difficulty Sleeping
- Irritability
- Tiredness

It's okay to feel a little sad after all that we've been through. Don't freak out if every once in a while, you start crying for no apparent reason. As common as it is to have a baby, it's truly a unique and extraordinary experience. Our bodies have been gearing up for childbirth for the last nine months, and within a few relatively short hours, it's all over. Think about it. We go to school for twelve-plus years, we graduate, and if you're anything like me, we still had no idea what is about to happen with our lives. Don't beat yourself up if you feel overwhelmed with the responsibility of taking care of an entirely dependent human being. Don't stress out if you feel like there isn't an instant bond between you and your baby, or that you don't feel overly excited about your baby right away. You may feel like a lousy mother because, for the first day or two, all you want to do is scarf down a cheeseburger and take a long nap. Let everyone around you be excited about the baby. I experienced all of these feelings and more. Don't worry; it's normal.

If, however, you feel like you're in a bottomless pit and can't get out, or you feel like checking into a hotel and never coming home, that's a different story. If you feel like you could do harm to yourself or your baby, get help immediately.

CHAPTER 8:

POSTPARTUM DEPRESSION (PPD)

Postpartum depression is something that you should talk about to loved ones. And then see a doctor. Seriously. The biggest problem with postpartum depression (PPD) is not dealing with it. If, for any reason, you find yourself isolated, especially as we experienced in 2020 during the COVID-19 pandemic, PPD can creep up and take hold of you.

Check out the website *findapsychologist.org*. Dr. Rosalind S. Dorlan, Psy.D., has a very informative article that explains PPD well, and I quote her:

"Despite the wonderful joy that a newborn can bring, the year following childbirth is actually the most vulnerable time for a woman to experience a mental health disorder, such as postpartum depression. Many factors may play a role, such as:

- Previous depression or postpartum depression
- First-time mothers
- A family history of mental illness
- A substance abuse history

- Complications at delivery
- Extreme sleep deprivation
- A very difficult or health-challenged baby
- Not enough support from family and friends
- High levels of stress."

I felt like I could check four out of nine from the list. PPD is a condition that can affect up to twenty-five percent of new mothers. Interestingly, it has also affected women who adopt a baby (*5-Minute Clinical Consult*, Lippincott, Williams & Wilkins). While most women experience some form of baby blues, not all new mothers with the blues will experience postpartum depression. It's important to distinguish between the two. PPD has several signs and symptoms that occur for at least two weeks straight. The US Department of Health and Social Services, on its website, lists the following feelings that may indicate a mother is suffering from PPD:

- Crying a lot, sadness, feelings of hopelessness, emptiness, or feeling isolated
- Guilt, feelings of worthlessness, or being a bad parent
- Exhaustion, extreme fatigue, low or no energy, no motivation
- Feeling anxious or having panic attacks

- Speech impairment, changes in movement and walking, sluggishness or restlessness
- Difficulty concentrating and making decisions
- Insomnia, or sleeping too much
- Eating disorders, sudden weight loss or weight gain and overeating
- Loss of pleasure in daily activities and in those around you
- Chronic headaches, aches and pains, or stomach upset
- Thoughts of harming yourself or thoughts of causing harm to the baby

If you experience such thoughts, I urge you to call a suicide hotline. In the US, call the National Suicide Prevention Lifeline at 1-800-273-TALK (1-800-273-8255) or use their webchat on *suicidepreventionlifeline.org/chat*.

A few weeks after returning home from the hospital, I felt completely alone. My in-laws had left. My husband was back at work, my family lived in another country, and my best friend was unable to visit because she'd just delivered a baby of her own. I'd taken twelve weeks of maternity leave from work and missed the camaraderie of my teammates. I felt isolated, and I was exhausted. I was up every two or three hours, day and night, breastfeeding my baby while dealing with the cramping of a shrinking uterus and the pain of an episiotomy incision that felt like the length of a small banana, although it was probably only a couple of centimeters long.

I started to think I had a case of the baby blues. Adding to my sense of inadequacy, my baby would scream, and I couldn't figure out why. At that time, we lived in a two-story house. My bedroom was across the hall from the nursery. The master bedroom was separated from the other bedrooms by a stairwell. Every time I crossed the aisle to comfort my screaming infant, the movie *Throw Momma from the Train* replayed in my brain. The film is about a son, played by Danny DeVito, who fantasizes about killing his overbearing mother. He enlists the help of his writing instructor, played by Billy Crystal, who pushes her from a moving train, only for her to be rescued by a repentant Danny DeVito. It made me feel incredibly guilty that I entertained thoughts of ending the crying by dropping my baby from the top of the stairwell. It got to a point where I looked away from the staircase every time I passed by. If I carried her from the nursery to my bedroom, I squeezed her extra tightly and deliberately made a path as far from the staircase as possible. I began to loathe the open space, which taunted me with a sheer drop of about twenty feet. I felt as though I couldn't share my thoughts with anyone, not even my husband. What if he called social services and they sent me away? What if he called the police and they arrested me? As much as motherhood was making me crazy, I didn't want to be away from my baby. Looking back, I felt inadequate and guilty because my baby wouldn't feed from my breast, I was exhausted, and I felt alone. As it appeared, I had experienced a touch of PPD.

Early detection of PPD is essential for the overall well-being of you and your newborn. If you think you're experiencing any of the signs, make a copy of the following questions and check off your symptoms. Have your partner, husband, friend, or relative help you with the list. Take this list to your doctor and talk about each category you checked and the frequency and intensity of those feelings. Go to your OB/GYN or your family doctor. Sometimes we can be so entrenched in our feelings that we don't realize we're suffering from a disease that a professional can quickly identify and treat. You're not alone. Your doctor will probably ask a few easy and straightforward questions. Answer the questions honestly; this isn't our driver's license (how many of us are honest about our height and weight?!).

Sometimes taking a self-test is helpful to determine what's going on, if anything. There are quite a few self-tests or quizzes on the internet, and most of the questions asked are similar in nature. The questions reflect how you've been feeling for the last seven days, not just at this particular moment. Below are a few questions from a postpartum self-test developed in Edinburgh, the Edinburgh Postnatal Depression Scale (EPDS).

Questions include things like:

1. I have been able to laugh and see the funny side of things (as much as I always could; not quite so much now; definitely not so much now; not at all)

2. I've looked forward with enjoyment to things

3. I have blamed myself unnecessarily when things went wrong

4. I have been anxious or worried for no good reason

5. I have felt scared or panicky for no good reason

6. Things have been getting on top of me

7. I have been so unhappy that I have had difficulty sleeping

8. I have felt sad or miserable

9. I have been so unhappy that I have been crying

10. The thought of harming myself has occurred to me (quite often, sometimes, hardly ever, never?)

There are many indications of PPD and many risk factors. It may not be the result of one item on a list. A little piece from multiple lists adds up to a lot. Take a good look at yourself with a partner, they may be able to see the things we can't see.

There is hope, and most PPD resolves reasonably quickly with a little help from either medication or psychotherapy, or both. Practical measures include getting adequate sleep and rest, a healthy diet, plenty of water for hydration, and keeping in mind the old adage, "Fresh air will do you a world of good." God help me; I'm hearing my mother's words of wisdom from when I was a child. "Go for a walk, run around the block, and soak up the sun. Eat a slice of bread. Try going to the bathroom." Seriously, stay away from caffeine, alcohol, and other drugs—unless recommended by your physician. Medications sometimes help.

Be completely honest with your physician about your feelings, and don't be afraid to say you may need a little help getting back to "normal."

Medications Your Doctor May Prescribe

Several medications may help—some increase chemical transmitters in the brain, such as serotonin, norepinephrine, or dopamine. The SSRIs (Selective Serotonin Reuptake Inhibitors) help increase serotonin levels, making us feel differently about our emotional responses. They include brand names such as Paxil (paroxetine), Prozac (fluoxetine), Zoloft (sertraline), and Celexa (citalopram). Some work on a combination of neurotransmitters, such as Wellbutrin and Aplenzin (bupropion), which increase serotonin and norepinephrine, mirtazapine (Remeron), and Effexor XR (venlafaxine). Treating depression is not an exact science, so be patient. Each person is different, and some mothers may do well on one medication, whereas other moms may need two or three medicines to get better. Your physician wants to hear about your feelings, and your physician is there to help.

CHAPTER 9:

ONE MORE STITCH, PLEASE! AND SEX AFTER PREGNANCY

That's right. My biggest fear going into pregnancy was having a vaginal birth and forever being stretched out down under. The thought of having a "wizard's sleeve" for a vagina was daunting. I ended up having an episiotomy and hoped my OB was generous with his sewing thread. I figured a couple of extra stitches couldn't hurt, right? A stitch for "daddy?" An additional "husband stitch"? At every prenatal visit, I let my OB know about my fear of having a vaginal birth and developing a "black hole" for a vagina, a vast nothingness that my husband would disappear into and never return. I would drop hints about a scheduled C-section and whether having one would be an option for me. I told him I wanted to avoid the legacy of a floppy vagina at all costs. Of course, a C-section, he informed me, was entirely out of the question as long as my pregnancy progressed normally and I had no complications during delivery. As for the "daddy" stitch, I'm so happy I had such an amazing OB who listened to my fears, sympathized, and ultimately possessed the medical skills, ethics, and experience to put the appropriate number of stitches between my vagina and my anus and no more. The "daddy stitch," I later discovered, is not recommended.

Usually, painful sex is the result of an extra stitch or two. That was the last thing I wanted. *Healthline.com* talks at length about this phenomenon, quoting OB/GYN Jesanna Cooper, M.D., who explains, "A 'husband stitch' would not affect overall vaginal tone, as this has much more to do with pelvic floor strength and integrity than introitus (opening) size."

Oh, so it's a muscle thing? Here we go again; I can't emphasize enough, Kegel, Kegel, Kegel, ladies! Another interesting tidbit from *Medical News Today*, and I'm quoting from medicalnewstoday.com, "A woman's vagina is almost never too tight to have sex. The pain or discomfort is a symptom of other issues (like the daddy stitch). In its unaroused state, the vagina is between three and four inches long and may not produce enough lubrication for comfortable intercourse. However, when aroused, the vagina expands in width and length and releases lubrication."

Huh, I had no idea that I'm a "grower" too!

The first time my husband and I became intimate after childbirth, I was scared to death. I had a million questions running through my head. Would I pop an episiotomy stitch?

How much would it hurt? Would I enjoy having sex again? How would my vagina feel to my husband? Had I Kegel'ed enough? Ah, I knew I should have Kegel'ed some more. Would my belly be an obstacle? Needless to say, I was stressed, anxious, and feeling a little guilty for not looking forward to having sex with my husband, especially since I'd cut him off a couple of weeks before delivering because I felt too big to assume the position.

We waited six weeks to get busy for the first time--after my postpartum checkup. It was painful in the beginning, and I was as dry as the Sahara Desert. The first jab felt sharp. My advice is to put on a Barry White or Marvin Gaye CD, go slow, and let your partner know to be gentle before the "sexual healing" begins. Make sure your vagina is fully aroused before the crucial moment; otherwise, you'll clench up like a salted slug. Use plenty of lubricants too. Something not too sticky, either; my favorite is Vagisil. It's a water-based lubricant, so it's less messy. It's a little harder to find than K-Y but well worth a good search of the drugstore shelves.

It turns out that I wasn't alone in feeling unprepared for sexual activity after having a baby. Postpartum sexual health can be challenging. A May 2018 study, in *BMC Pregnancy and Childbirth*, by Dierdre O'Malley et al. reported that almost half of the 832 women studied experienced sexual health issues six months postpartum, while forty percent still had issues twelve months postpartum. Here's the breakdown:

- 46.3 percent reported a lack of interest in sex at six months
- 43 percent reported a lack of vaginal lubrication at six months
- 37.5 percent reported painful intercourse at six months

Several factors played a role in the lack of interest and the dryness of the vagina, including breastfeeding. This is not surprising since estrogen levels drop drastically during breastfeeding. We need estrogen to boost blood flow to our genitals and increase vaginal lubrication. Estrogen also helps with increased elasticity and thickness of the vaginal lining. *Healthline.com* reports that twenty-four hours after delivery, our estrogen drops to pre-pregnancy levels. Our bodies also produce prolactin and oxytocin during breastfeeding, which blocks estrogen production; both of these hormones can make us feel pleasure from feeding our baby, so who needs a partner? Just saying.

As a new mother adapting to motherhood, I was also dealing with lack of sleep; I wasn't happy with my body's size and shape; I was afraid our baby might wake up and start screaming once we got going; and my nipples hurt like hell. Not a good recipe for a long-overdue sexual encounter—sorry, partner! In all seriousness, the O'Malley et al. study stresses the need for new parents to be forewarned of the potential changes in postpartum sexual health. It may take a while for the dust to settle and for things to get back to normal, so having a discussion about each other's fears and waiting for the right time may be the best way forward.

CHAPTER 10:

SWEATING LIKE A PIG

This was another postpartum bodily function I wasn't prepared for—sweating like a pig! I thought there was something wrong with me when my muumuu of a nightgown was noticeably damp every morning, and the hair on the back of my neck was sopping wet. There appeared to be no accounting for my constant perspiration. It wasn't like I could move fast enough to work up a sweat; how could I? I was in constant fear of the subway sandwich slipping out of my undies. I had a cramp in my abdomen thanks to my shrinking uterus, and my undercarriage was sewn up so tightly that I squeaked when I moved. I couldn't understand it. Why was I sweating so much? Was I sick? Was my episiotomy incision infected? Was I going through "The Change?" I was in my early forties, after all. But wait, that would mean my daughter would be an only child. My husband and I both wanted two or three children. We're both from large families, and growing up, we enjoyed the noise, bickering, and chaos that comes with having multiple siblings. How could I break the news to my husband? Would he want to adopt? Could we afford adoption? How do I feel about adopting? With no concrete answers to all of the questions swirling through my mind, I singlehandedly upped my anxiety to yet another level.

I convinced myself that having a baby in my forties screwed with my hormones, and now I was going through menopause. I thought I was sweating profusely because I'd triggered "The Change." The internet confirmed my diagnosis with multiple websites that spelled out the symptoms of menopause: "Irregular periods, night sweats, chills, hot flashes, sleep disturbances." I had all of them, especially the hot flashes and night sweats. Everything was sweaty. My crotch was sweaty; my armpits were sweaty. My back was sweaty; the backs of my knees were slimy and sweaty; heck, my whole body was a ball of sweat. Nighttime was the worst. I would wake up two or three times from night sweats, and still have to get up to go pee. I needed to know how I would break the news to my husband. And I had to find the right moment.

A few weeks after delivering my first baby, I was excited to get myself gussied up and leave the house to attend a party at a friend's house. I was so happy to have something different to look forward to other than the usual; you know, wearing baggy sweatpants, milk-stained t-shirts, hair in a messy ponytail, and generally looking scruffy and unkempt. I had a goal—to shower, style my hair, and put on makeup. YAY! My tummy and my clothes still made me look pregnant; I couldn't get around that. But three out of four ain't bad. I was feeling quite good about myself and headed to the party. So, there I was, having a glass of wine (just one, because I was breastfeeding) and feeling like a normal person for a minute when a friend asked me about my baby. I spoke proudly of my little one, as any new mother would. I lamented that she would be my "one and only," and I felt sad and anxious about not having the opportunity to have more children. I explained my menopausal situation and told her I was experiencing the worst hot flashes and night sweats. She very abruptly stopped me and said, "You're breastfeeding!"

Wait, what?!

The same menopausal-like symptoms plagued her with each of her three babies while she was breastfeeding. She'd wake up blazing hot in the middle of the night and would find herself lying in a pool of sweat. She'd smack her husband to turn on the overhead fan for her. Then she'd be shivering because of the cold, wet jammies she was wearing. It was a vicious cycle—hot, cold, hot, cold. So, what to do?

A few days later, I called my best friend, who was at home on maternity leave with her second baby, and I'm so thankful I talked to her. She gave me some comforting news about my situation. She reminded me of how I looked during the last few weeks of pregnancy. I had so much water retention I looked as though I'd overdosed on steroids. Seriously, my face was as round as a full moon at night. I could hardly recognize my poor feet because they looked like footballs with five little stubs attached. I could press my finger into the skin around my ankle, and it would take thirty minutes for the indent to clear. Ridiculous!

The time had come for the additional fluid to exit my body as sweat and pee. As if I really wanted to add "more laundry" to my to-do list. I didn't have the time nor the patience for extra trips to the bathroom either, especially during the night, when all I wanted to do was sleep between feedings.

Postpartum sweating can last for a few weeks, and it's completely normal. It may last longer for women who breastfeed, and the reason seems to point to an obvious culprit—estrogen, yet again. After we have a baby and we're breastfeeding, our estrogen levels drop so low they're similar to the levels experienced by menopausal women. Breastfeeding women produce prolactin and tend to have lower levels of estrogen than women who feed exclusively from the bottle using baby formula. Prolactin is needed to produce breast milk, and prolactin also keeps estrogen levels low.

It will help if you stay hydrated during this time. It may

sound counterintuitive, but the more water you drink, the faster the elimination will be. So don't be tempted to skimp on your fluid intake. Another good reason to stay hydrated is to help ensure you have an adequate milk supply for your baby. Fill the most oversized cup you can find and make sure there's plenty of ice, water, a straw, and a tight lid. Carry it around with you like it's a second child. After giving birth, my parting gift from the hospital was a thirty-six-ounce, thick plastic cup with a plastic straw and a lid adorned with the hospital logo. The hospital had the sides of the mug printed with the words "101 Ways to Praise Your Child" and included terms of positive reinforcement such as "good job," "hot dog," and "you're unique." I made sure that puppy was iced up, full of water, and never more than an arm's length away. I was happy the lid had a secure fit because I was continually dropping the darned thing. One way to tell if you're getting enough water is to look at the color of your pee. If it's pale and there's plenty of it, you should be okay, but if it's dark yellow and scant, buck up and drink some more.

My friend suggested I sleep on a towel to cut down on the number of times I had to change the bedsheets. She was right; the towel soaked up most of the sweat and provided a second line of defense just in case the subway sandwich happened to spring a leak.

Some other ideas include sleeping in the nude—except, of course, for the granny panties, subway sandwich, support bra, and belly band. Let the air circulate as much as you can. If you have a houseful of guests popping in and out of the bedroom, wear loose-fitting, cotton nighties or jammies. Sleep with a fan on at night. If you don't have an overhead fan or a portable fan to put on your nightstand, open a window. If it's one hundred degrees outside and the humidity is ninety percent, don't open a window. If you feel super-hot, check your temperature, and call your doctor if the thermometer reads 100.4 degrees or more—you may have a fever, so you'll need a professional opinion.

CHAPTER 11

HAIR LOSS

While I was pregnant with my first baby, I remember going to a new hair salon, sitting in the chair, and trying to explain why the front of my hair looked like I'd cut out chunks of chewing gum. I had very obvious clumps of short hair that sat at the top of my forehead, right along my hairline. I couldn't hide it. The hair stuck straight up, looking a little ridiculous next to the rest of my long, straight locks. What had happened? I toyed with the idea that my previous hairdresser had overprocessed my hair while she was highlighting, or that I'd snapped off a wad every time I used a flat iron to straighten my hair. My hairdresser calmly explained that she came across the chewing-gum-stuck-in-the-hair look all the time; it was new hair growth because of pregnancy.

According to *babycenter.com*, a woman usually sheds about one hundred hairs a day—the majority of them fall out while we're brushing or washing our hair. If your hair is long like mine, it may appear as though you lose more than that, but it's only because long hair is more visible than short hair.

On any given day, eighty-five to ninety-five percent of our hair is in a "growing stage," which can last for up to seven years. The remaining five to fifteen percent is in a "resting stage," which lasts for about two to three months, after which, our hair falls out. New hair grows in its place, et voila, the average growth cycle of hair.

During pregnancy and nursing, things change thanks to, you guessed it, our hormones. Increased estrogen during pregnancy causes our hair to remain in the growing stage longer, which means fewer hairs are advancing to the resting stage and falling out. The result is a thicker head of hair because fewer hairs are shedding. As our estrogen levels drop after delivery, our hair graduates to the resting stage, and we all know what that means—next comes the falling-out stage. Suddenly, we lose those beautiful extra locks. Sometimes the hair falls out in clumps and clogs up the drain while shampooing. Mine would fall out in handfuls like I had a serious case of alopecia. It's normal; don't freak out. The worst for me was finding clumps of hairs in my bra or down the back of my t-shirt, making me itch like I had a bad case of fleas.

During pregnancy, my hair also took another strange turn. It went from straight to wavy, and eleven years after my first baby, it still hasn't returned to its pre-pregnancy straight look. I use a flat iron to straighten my hair nowadays. Most websites will say that our hair should return to its normal state of affairs within a year of giving birth and that permanently going from straight to curly or curly to straight is a rare occurrence. I should buy a lottery ticket—I must be part of the rare crowd! *Community.babycenter.com* surveyed women about how, or if, their hair changed after having babies. Out of forty-seven votes, nine women said their hair went from straight to wavy/curly, six went from wavy/curly to straight, and thirty-two said nope, their hair stayed the same. So, who knows what your hair will be like once you deliver? You may have a new hairdo and be pleasantly surprised!

CHAPTER 12:

AUNT FLO

So the baby's growing, she's putting on weight, and the delivery is becoming a distant memory. All is good. Then, two or three weeks after you stop breastfeeding, Aunt Flo comes for a visit. Just when you thought the sandwich in your panties was history!

Wow! Nobody thought to tell me to stock up on a ridiculously large supply of super-plus tampons and panty pads—not the liners, the full-on maternity pads. Before pregnancy, I was a regular-sized tampon girl with the very occasional need for the odd super here and there. I'd never handled a super-plus before! Once Aunt Flo arrived, I started to go through tampons and pads like a kid going through candy on Halloween night.

I wouldn't call the visits periods; they were "bleeds." Each one would last about five days and, for each of those days, whenever I left the house, I scouted the nearest bathroom location, just in case I needed a quick change. Like the first few weeks after delivery, I found myself popping a clean pair

of panties into my purse whenever I left the house in prepara-
tion for the inevitable. My handbag became a portable storage
chest for a plethora of disposable menstrual products. With
so many supplies, I feared the idea of standing in the checkout line at my local grocery store and opening my purse to
have a collection of giant super-plus tampons pop out on the
conveyor belt. An article by Chella Quint, published in *inde-
pendent.co.uk* in October 2017, talks about matching our
products to our handbags, belts, and shoes. She calls it "vajaz-
zling." Not a bad idea, especially for the accidental handbag
spillage!

Emma-Louise Pritchard wrote an article for *Cospomoli-
tan.com/uk*, published in March 2016, in which she talks about
how women refer to their periods by terms other than "period." She says women worldwide use alternate names to de-
scribe their period seventy-eight percent of the time. There
are the obvious ones: Monthly Visitor, Red Tide, On the Rag,
Riding the Crimson Tide, and the most descriptive for our initial postpartum period, Shark Week.

Why is it not surprising that young girls often feel socially
awkward about periods when seventy-eight percent of the
time adults feel embarrassed to use the term "period"? Add to
that the fact that most of us start our period while we're still
children, and add menstrual cramps, numerous trips to the

bathroom, and the fear of sudden movements causing leakage; it's a lot for a girl to deal with each month. Girls are unintentionally trained to feel less confident from an early age. In school, we skulk around trying to hide the fact we're on our period. Why don't boys in school get the period talk too? Why don't boys go through some sort of a period awareness class and wear thick pads in their undies to gain understanding? Maybe they'd be more sympathetic? Maybe girls would be more confident for an additional five days every month. Just a thought.

My first postpartum period started about eleven weeks after delivery, and, initially, the frequency was pretty erratic. My second postpartum period followed two weeks after the first, and then they followed every three to four weeks after that. One of my friends had it worse than I. After her first postpartum period, another bloodbath followed about a week later. Her periods remained heavy for a number of years. She eventually had an ablation procedure to help her situation. It wasn't until my seventh period, around thirty-two weeks postpartum, that my flow became normal—lucky seven! I couldn't believe I was back to using regular tampons, thank God! During this time, I discovered a surprising benefit to wearing tampons—for five days a month, I had better bladder control. As long as I was wearing a tampon, I could cough without a major incident; I could run, jump, and have a good old belly laugh without the need to excuse myself for an underwear change.

Okay, I can't leave this chapter without coming back to some international references for our time of the month. Emma-Louise Pritchard, in her *Cosmopolitan* piece, also lists colloquial names from around the world. Here goes, and I'm quoting:

1. The Communists Are in the Funhouse (Denmark)
2. The English Have Landed (France)
3. Mad Cow Disease (Finland)
4. Granny's Stuck in Traffic (South Africa)
5. I'm with Chico (Brazil)
6. The Cranberry Woman Is Coming (Germany)

Clue.com states there are more than 5,000 euphemisms around the world for "period," including:

1. France - Grumbling; The Carrots Are Cooked; The Beaujolais Nouveau Wine Has Arrived
2. Italy - I Have My Things; The Marques; I Have a Flood
3. Japan - The Arrival of Commodore Matthew Perry; The Monthly Things; and Girl's Day

SECTION THREE

CHAPTER 13

BLADDER CONTROL, OR NOT

One day, early in my pregnancy, I caught an ABC sitcom episode of *The Middle.* During the show, mom and dad (played by Patricia Heaton and Neil Flynn) facilitated sibling bonding by playing a game of touch football as a family. Their three children were on one team, and mom and dad were on the opposing team—children versus adults. The children had an ace in the hole, not only because their parents were tired, out of shape, and middle-aged, but because mom and dad each had a handicap. During the huddle, Axl, the oldest son, explained to his teammates that "Dad's peripheral vision is going, and Mom can't run too fast, or she'll pee."

No way, I thought. But after having kids, I can totally relate. Once my doctor gave me the nod at my six-week checkup to exercise and go back to normal activities, I noticed I peed at the slightest body movement. When I laughed, I peed. When I picked up my baby or lifted a stack of plates from the dishwasher, I whizzed. If I reached to catch a ball or hoisted a heavy bag of groceries, I dribbled. Any sudden movement caused me to tinkle in my drawers.

When my daughter was about three years old, I had a horrendous sinus infection that took two rounds of antibiotics to clear up. As the mucus started to break up and drain down my throat, it sent me into fits of coughing, followed by uncontrollable bladder squirts. I remember the day the US women's soccer team won a crucial game in the World Cup. The US defeated Norway one-nill in the quarterfinals. My daughter and I jumped off the couch and into the air with excitement. As my arms reached for the stars in celebration, my legs dribbled with pee from my leaking bladder. I experienced incident after incident. I have so many vivid memories indelibly etched in my brain, not because of the occasion itself but because of the anxiety I suffered from concluding an event with a wet leg and a soggy crotch.

Probably the worst accident happened while I was pregnant with my second child. It was something I'll never forget. I was almost at the end of my first trimester when I came down with another stuffy head cold. I was concerned about taking medications known to harm a growing baby, so my safe options were few and far between—no more Mucinex, Benadryl, or codeine. I had to deal with severe nasal and head congestion without my go-to medication. On vacation, while in the beautiful city of Seville, Spain, I was enjoying a fun day of sightseeing when it hit me like a ton of bricks. I felt a tickle in the back of my throat, and I started to cough uncontrollably.

My face got red, my eyes started watering, and I coughed so hard I could hardly breathe. I felt like I was going to throw up. That's when I noticed pee flowing down my leg. My panty liner couldn't hold it anymore; as Scotty would say on board the original USS *Enterprise*, "She's gonna blow, Captain!" And then she blew. All I could do was sit down on the sidewalk and wait for it to be over. I needed a bathroom desperately. But I couldn't move. Finally, I caught my breath and found myself sitting in a pool of warm urine. My wonderful husband dried my eyes and helped me stand up. I'd soiled myself from my underwear down to my shoes, and my chest was sore from coughing so hard. My husband grabbed a wad of napkins from a curbside food vendor, and that's what I used to dry myself off. I was in such a sorry state—red-faced, covered in pee, and feeling utterly embarrassed and defeated. All I wanted to do was make my way back to the solace and safety of the condominium where we were staying, escape from the world, and take a nice, hot, relaxing bath. Oh, that's right; I'm pregnant, NO HOT BATHS!

Yep, I'm discovering I'm turning into my mother. Growing up, I would accompany her to the grocery store, and I noticed she would frequently drop a packet of thick, bulky panty pads into the shopping cart. She kept a bountiful supply in her dresser drawer, even after menopause. My mother would always cross her legs when she needed to sneeze or cough. I could never understand why. Now it all makes sense. She gave birth to three singles and a set of twins, all vaginal and in the 1950s and '60s. No wonder she experienced postpartum bladder leakage. She, like millions of other women around the world, was living with urinary incontinence.

My urinary incontinence became so problematic that several years after delivering I still found myself carrying an extra pair of underwear in my purse. I wouldn't think of leaving the house without a heavy-duty panty liner firmly glued to my gusset, in addition to a stash hidden in my handbag. It got to the point that even when taking a gentle stroll for exercise, I would experience leakage. Any rigorous activity was utterly out of the question. How would I lose those extra pounds if I couldn't move faster than a snail? And sadly, like a snail, I would occasionally leave a trail behind after exerting myself.

Why does no one talk about this? Think about how prevalent urinary incontinence is and how many women live with decreased mobility because they're fearful of making sudden movements. Think about how many women live with shame from peeing themselves thanks to an innocent sneeze, cough, or belly laugh. The Norwegian Mother and Child Cohort Study, published in 2009, concluded that as many as thirty-one per-cent of new mothers experience urinary incontinence at six months postpartum. The bladder control industry is a billion-dollar-a-year money-making business because the condition is so common. Store shelves are full of different products claiming to help women manage urinary incontinence. There are panty liners, panty pads, disposable underwear (don't think I haven't tried them), non-disposable undergarments, adult diapers, and waterproof bed sheets. Who hasn't heard of Depend bladder control pads? Watch the evening news shows, and commercials pop up offering to deliver them discreetly to your home in a plain cardboard box. There are also medical devices available to help control bladder leaks. They include catheters, pessaries, guards, barrier devices, and products worn inside the vagina, products that work outside the vagina, muscle stimulators, and prescription drugs. Who knew?

STRESS INCONTINENCE

Needless to say, one of the risk factors for stress urinary incontinence is vaginal childbirth.

If you were an "Assisted Vaginal Delivery," which means your doctor or midwife used forceps or a vacuum device, you're even more at risk. Maybe you had a large baby, or, like me, you have a small pelvic opening, and the forceps were essentially the hands of a doctor; well, we're also more at risk. Some women who've had C-sections experience leakage from stress incontinence, but fewer C-section moms experience this than moms who delivered vaginally. The Norwegian Mother and Child Cohort Study cited forceps delivery, vacuum delivery, and age as the most common reasons for urinary incontinence six months after delivery. For most women, the condition only lasts for a few months, but it can be a lifelong affliction for others, including myself.

The most common cause of urinary stress incontinence during pregnancy is extra pressure on the bladder. As a result, the bladder sphincter can't do its job properly and allows pee to escape. Activities such as coughing and sneezing provide a temporary bolt of pressure that completely overpowers the sphincter and, as in my case, squirts pee down my leg like a pastry chef piping frosting on a Bundt cake. Bladder compression can result from the uterus's weight sitting on top, extra body weight, or full bowels from constipation.

During delivery, the bladder can become overstretched or damaged. The ligaments holding up the bladder can be damaged or become detached. Pushing the baby can strain or weaken the pelvic floor muscles and/or the nerves surrounding the bladder. The bladder could prolapse or fall out of position. And let's not forget those pesky hormone changes, especially with relaxin, that cause joints and support tissue in the pelvis to relax, decreasing support for the bladder and making it more difficult for us to control the stream.

The answer?

The first line of therapy recommended by most medical communities is the old pelvic floor muscle therapy. You guessed it—Kegel, Kegel, and Kegel. And just when you thought you were Kegel'ed out, Kegel some more, please!

Unfortunately, Kegel'ing day and night did little for me. In the name of research and the pursuit of dry panties, I decided to investigate how I could control my stress incontinence. It took seven years from my first delivery to ask my OB/GYN about my condition. I plucked up the nerve to talk about it during my annual checkup. My OB/GYN took a good look and told me it appeared I had a detached ligament; nothing too serious. Huh, he could see that from just looking up there during an exam? Amazing. He gave me the contact information of a couple of experts in the fields of urology and urogynecology, a surgical subspecialty.

I made an appointment for a consult. On the day of my meeting, I was nervous but hopeful. After checking in with the receptionist, the doctor invited me into his office for a quick chat. He talked with me for about ten to fifteen minutes, and asked all kinds of questions about how often I peed, what triggered my peeing, and how much pee did I pee when I peed. Quite a tongue-twister! After gathering his information, he walked me into an exam room. It was time for me to strip from the waist down, put on a gown, and lay down on the examination table. I scooched down, put my feet in the stirrups, and relaxed my buttock muscles. We're all familiar with the drill. After another quick examination, he inserted his finger and asked me to clench my pelvic floor muscles as hard as I could. It felt a little awkward, but okay. After a hard squeeze, he told me my pelvic floor muscles appeared intact and they were still strong. My OB/GYN was right; I had a slightly detached ligament. Phew! I had a diagnosis.

The doctor then left the exam room to allow me to put on my clothes. Once dressed, I returned to his office and sat down for another quick chat. He sat across the desk from me and told me I'd make an excellent candidate for bladder sling surgery. He explained my diagnosis by telling me to picture a garden hose lying on a stable concrete path. If everything worked as it should, I'd be able to step on the hose and stop the flow of water. My ligament represented the concrete path, and it was detached. Without the simultaneous pressure from underneath, water would leak from the hose regardless of how much pressure I exerted. My detached ligament was like a crumbling concrete walkway, unable to exert enough pressure to stop the water flow.

So now I knew what I was dealing with, and I also knew that no matter how many Kegels I practiced, I would leak. I felt better knowing that my condition could be fixed with surgery, and that help lay just around the corner.

My doctor explained the procedure. Since he couldn't re-attach my ligament, he would insert a mesh strip into my body to act as a sling to support my urethra (the tube that transports pee from the bladder to the outside of the body). My mind started whirling. How would he insert it? Would the mesh be made of metal? Would it trigger the metal detectors at the airport, and if it did set off the sensors, what would I say to the security officer? "I'm not packing, honest! It's just an innocent strip of metal holding up my bladder to prevent me from peeing all over the airport floor. Really!"

The surgeon sensed my anxiety. Maybe it was the look of horror on my face?! He pushed a brochure across the desk in hopes of calming me. The leaflet contained detailed information about the mesh. In addition, my doctor explained that the type of mesh he used for bladder sling surgery is made from synthetic material. No metal—a potentially embarrassing metal detector situation averted.

My doctor told me the type of surgery best suited for my situation was called retropubic sling surgery, and he broke it down for me. He'd make a small incision inside my vagina, just below my urethra. He'd also make a couple of small incisions in my pubic area, just above my hairline. With a needle threaded with synthetic mesh, he'd start sewing by inserting the needle into one of the pubic area incisions, and then head down to the vagina. The mesh in the needle would act as a hammock to support my urethra. He'd make a few stitches in the vagina to hold the mesh in place, then come back up and out of the incision on the other side of the pubic area. In, down, stitch, up, and out. He'd use dissolving stitches so I wouldn't have to go back and have stitches removed. The recovery would involve rest, nothing in the hoo-ha for six weeks (sounds familiar), and no heavy lifting. The good news was that my health insurance would cover the cost of the procedure, so I didn't have to worry about the financial aspect of the surgery.

According to *clevelandclinic.org*, as many as 250,000 women in the US underwent bladder sling surgery in 2010, and 300,000 women had surgery to fix a pelvic organ prolapse (PPP). Pregnancy, childbirth, and age are the most common factors causing PPP, and the result can be bladder leakage, pain, and discomfort. Weakened or overstretched pelvic floor muscles are unable to support the pelvic organs. More commonly it's the bladder that prolapses, but other organs include the uterus, rectum, vagina, and urethra that fall downward and bulge out of the vagina. It can easily be diagnosed with a pelvic exam.

I wrestled with the idea of having an operation and of inserting mesh into my body. Could I afford the recovery time, six weeks? And would it really work?

I took to the internet and started researching. I came across an article from *babycentre.co.uk* with the headline, *"Stress incontinence isn't something you should just accept as a normal part of being a mum. It could affect your mental health if you continue to leak, so don't wait to get help."* I thought about the amount of weight I'd gained in the last seven years, and about how I wasn't able to exercise without peeing myself. I thought about Kristen Bell in the movie *Bad Moms*. She played an overworked, underappreciated mom named Kiki, who fantasized about getting into a car wreck (nothing major) so she could have a few days in the hospital to escape from her kids crawling all over her. All she wanted was to relish in the luxury of staying in bed and watching TV all day. And then I thought about how nice it would be to have time to myself with no interruptions. "Doctor's Orders!" I decided it was time for bladder sling surgery.

CHAPTER 14

BLADDER SLING SURGERY

Once I'd made up my mind to have the surgical "fix," I could hardly wait. All I could think about was life without squirting in my skivvies. I'd chalked up seven years of diligently wearing panty liners. A liner or a pad every single day, some days changing them two or three times. Let's do the math—seven years multiplied by one liner multiplied by 365 days. That equals a minimum of 2,555 soiled panty liners from laughing too hard, sneezing too hard, running after, and picking up chubby little kids. Could the panty liner industry survive without me?

Finally, the big day arrived. The procedure was quick, relatively painless, and life-changing. The surgery itself took around thirty minutes. It took longer to check into the outpatient center and prep for surgery than the surgery itself. After I awoke from anesthesia, I found myself in a comfortable bed with warm blankets, and I relished the attention of multiple professionals taking care of me. My nurses were great. My doctor sent me home armed with several prescriptions; one was for a week of narcotics, OxyContin; another for a week of

NSAIDs, ibuprofen; and a third for a stool softener, Dulcolax. The last thing I wanted to do was pop a stitch straining from a bowel movement!

The recovery was a breeze. My pubic area was swollen and purple from bruising. I sported two small circles, one on each side, that were colored with a smidge of red blood. My pubic area looked as if a giant rattlesnake had bitten me. Of course, I milked the situation by having my family wait on me hand and foot. It was marvelous! I only needed to take the narcotics for a couple of days after surgery. Overall, the pain was manageable. Ibuprofen helped with the uncomfortable twinges here and there. The hardest part of my recovery was that I couldn't lift anything, which meant I couldn't pick up my little one. She was almost two years old, and she couldn't understand why I wasn't reaching down to slip my arms under her and pull her in for a cuddle. It was heartbreaking hearing her emulate Peppa Pig by repeating "Mommy Ig?" and looking down at her puzzled face, her arms up in the air, "Up, pweeze." Who doesn't watch the adorable Peppa Pig when you have a little one?

The best part about bladder sling surgery is that it has a ninety-percent success rate. And the best part about my recovery was lying in bed, uninterrupted for hours on end, catching up on Netflix and grown-up TV shows. I was very fortunate that everything was successful. If you don't need to go the surgery route, here are some tips that may help worn-out pelvic floor muscles.

HELPFUL TIPS TO CONTROL BLADDER LEAKAGE

- Try to get in three sets of thirty Kegel exercises a day.
- The closer you are to your ideal weight, the easier it will be to control your situation, because those extra pounds are still putting pressure on your bladder. The chicken and the egg, right? You can't exercise if you pee; you need to exercise to lose weight and curb the pee.
- Train your bladder. Try to urinate every thirty minutes, regardless of whether you have the urge or not, and then extend the time between bathroom visits each day. Also, try stopping the flow midstream and hold it for a second or two, then finish.
- Try to avoid constipation after pregnancy; that way, full bowels don't put added pressure on your bladder.
- Try to drink at least eight glasses of water every day (cutting back on drinking water to control the peeing only makes you susceptible to dehydration and urinary tract infections).

- Caffeine may aggravate the situation because it increases urine volume and can irritate the bladder itself. So, in essence, cut down on caffeine-containing foods and drinks such as coffee, chocolate (:-(sad face), and also citrus, tomatoes, and alcohol—all of which can aggravate your bladder and make peeing harder to control.
- Wear panty pads or panty liners to help absorb leaking urine and prevent an embarrassing wet spot. Surprisingly, I found that wearing a tampon helped, but I wouldn't recommend wearing one every day.

As a last line of defense, do Kegels or cross your legs when you feel the need to cough, sneeze, laugh, or lift something heavy.

CHAPTER 15:

WITCHY NAILS, SKIN TAGS & OTHER SOUVENIRS OF PREGNANCY

WITCHY NAILS

I don't have to be a detective or play Magnum P.I. to spot a new mom. There are so many subtle, telltale signs, and I'm not just referring to the nearby baby stroller, the milk-stained t-shirt, or the crossing of her legs at the onset of a sneeze.

One of the subtler badges of motherhood may be vertical ridges on her nails. I used to have silky-smooth nails until I became pregnant. Then I noticed my thumbnails changing. They became grooved and developed ridges in the nail bed as they grew. My thumbnails looked like they were housing a fungus infection. Hoping this was another one of those temporary hormonal changes, I figured my nails would straighten up after the baby was born and return to their pre-pregnancy silky-smooth texture.

Years later, I'm still waiting for this to happen. My friends told me my nails would grow faster during pregnancy—because of the extra blood volume and increased hormones. They'd say to me, "Enjoy your long nails and pamper yourself with manicures." Little did I know that nails can also become brittle and weak during this time, which also means they can be damaged easily.

I hadn't owned a nail brush before pregnancy. Growing up, we had one in our family bathroom. My father was the only one in our household who used it. He was an engineer and enjoyed working in his home workshop, creating playsets for our backyard. Sometimes, before dinner, he'd work on vehicle engines and needed a nail brush to scrub the oil and dirt from his fingernails. During pregnancy, I needed a nail brush; only I didn't need one for cleaning behind my nails. Instead, I needed one to scrub the surface of my nails. The ridges were so prominent they gathered dirt and debris. I now have to file the tips of my thumbnails and the entire nail bed because the crinkles still haven't grown out.

Typically, when vertical ridges, white spots, or black spots appear on our fingernails during pregnancy, they disappear about three to six months after delivery. It may take nine to twelve months for our toenails to return to normal. Many websites and medical community members say changes in our nails' appearance can occur at any time, not only during pregnancy. Some changes can be a sign of a possible health concern.

www.mayoclinic.org is a great website that outlines some health conditions associated with variations in fingernails, and, best of all, there are pictures.

Who doesn't like to ogle photos of crazy nail or skin conditions? *Skinsight.com* says our fingernails typically grow 0.1 millimeters (mm) per day, and our toenails grow about 0.03 mm per day (maybe faster during pregnancy). Problems with our nails' appearance may be due to many complications, including trauma to the nail bed, a mineral or vitamin deficiency (especially during pregnancy), vascular disease, stress, or kidney disease. Vertical lines, which are typically harmless, may also prevail after delivery because of advancing age. Check! Hmmm, maybe I should mention my thumbnails to my doctor the next time I go for a checkup, just to be on the safe side.

SKIN TAGS

Another result of pregnancy, which, by the way, was somewhat comforting to me because it reminded me of my late father, was the sudden emergence of skin tags. They resembled small rice grains that stood straight up, and, much like surprise lilies, they appeared from nowhere. For the most part, they were the same color as the majority of my skin, although some of them were a few shades darker. They especially liked to grow in the folds of my skin. They appeared in my armpits, under my breasts, neck, and in my groin area. They grew in places where my skin rubbed together. I found a slew of them under my breasts, large ones, tiny ones, and, in some areas, they appeared in clusters. I ended up with way too many of them to count. They seemed to breed like rabbits, especially during my second and third trimesters. I suppose they were inevitable because I carried plenty of extra weight. By the end of my pregnancy, my skin rubbed together almost everywhere.

But there's no need to freak out about them. They're entirely benign, and, yes, it's widely believed they appear due to increased hormones and weight gain. Our skin's outer layer is hyperactive during pregnancy because it needs to grow to cover our expanding belly. Leptin is released from fat tissue during pregnancy and also from the growing fetus. It can cause the growth of epithelial skin cells (the outer layer of our skin), and leptin can drive the growth of skin tags.

If, after delivery, they bother you, you could see your doctor or dermatologist. A medical professional can freeze them off, numb them and cut them off, or cauterize them. Be leery of some home remedies to remove them that you read about on the internet. Harsh ingredients can irritate the skin. After pregnancy, they usually shrivel up and fall off by themselves. Sometimes the stubborn ones remain. I had one on my back where my bra closure snapped together, and it rubbed and rubbed as I moved. It was so sore. I asked my husband to clip it off with a pair of scissors, but he couldn't bring himself to do it. I offered him nail clippers. He still couldn't bring himself to do it. He was convinced it would hurt me. I'd already tried clipping off the ones I could reach and discovered that, although cutting them wasn't painful, they can bleed, so be careful.

A couple of years after pregnancy, I'd had enough of twisting my arm around my back to scratch the skin tag under my bra snap. I made an appointment with my dermatologist to see what she could do. She took care of it in minutes—clip, and it was gone. The stubborn skin tags under my breasts don't bother me; they're so small I hardly notice them, but I was so thankful to have the pesky one on my back removed once and for all!

PREGNANCY MASK

I have a twin brother who has continually made fun of my forehead ever since I became pregnant for the first time. My forehead looked like I was wearing a speckled brown mask. My skin became mottled with patches of light brown here and specks of dark brown there; it looked like an abstract painting worthy of hanging in an art museum. My babies are summer babies; one arrived in June, and my other baby arrived at the end of July. Both of those summers were scorching hot and sunny. My job at the time involved popping in and out of offices all day, which meant I spent about two hours a day in full sun. My Northern European skin doesn't handle the sun well, even at the best of times. Fluctuating hormones and blazing sunshine during pregnancy sent my delicate facial skin into a flummox. While pregnant, I was cautious of using retinol creams or bleaching creams; all I could do was slather my face with factor-50 sunscreen. I continued slapping on the sunscreen well after my deliveries. Only my mask stayed strong. It didn't fade.

I discovered I belong to the "lucky" ten percent of women in whom melasma, chloasma, or pregnancy mask persists after delivery. Birth control pills can also cause the "mask of pregnancy," thanks to changing hormones. I was lucky it appeared only on my forehead and not all over my face; I could use a coverup cream and makeup in just one area. I tried several home remedies that didn't help, including apple cider vinegar, tomato paste, and black tea water. I experimented like an owner of a skunked dog, trying every urban legend remedy to eradicate the mask of pregnancy. (FYI, to eliminate the smell of skunk spray, try mixing a bottle of hydrogen peroxide with a few tablespoons of baking soda and a few drops of dish soap. It works).

I also tried expensive store-shelf creams, to no avail. Then a friend told me to try a prescription-strength hydroquinone cream. I called my dermatologist's office, made an annual skin check appointment, and walked out of the office with a prescription for Tri-Luma. It contained twice the strength of hydroquinone found in over-the-counter creams, (used to lighten dark spots) along with a corticosteroid (to reduce skin inflammation), and tretinoin (like retinol to reduce dark spots and strengthen the skin). I was pretty excited to give it a go.

I applied the cream every evening before bedtime, and my pregnancy mask was hardly noticeable in a matter of weeks. It was like a miracle cream. To this day, eleven years later, I remain vigilant about applying sunscreen all over my face because, in blazing sunshine, my mask reappears, albeit to a lesser extent. Thanks, pregnancy hormones!

STRETCH MARKS

Like mother, like daughter. Stretch marks (or striae gravidarum) have a genetic component. If you come from a gene pool of women with very elastic skin, chances are you're one of the lucky few who avoids the stretch mark scars of pregnancy. Unfortunately, I'm one of the ninety percent of women who end up with annoying permanent tear marks from overstretched skin. I considered myself lucky, given the amount of weight I piled on during my first pregnancy. I only developed a few on the underside of my belly and on the sides of my breasts. There's a train of thought that older women, whose skin is looser than younger women, fare better because taut, youthful skin is already very tight before the "Big Stretch" of pregnancy. Older skin has a little more room to give.

Some women keep their skin supple and hydrated with oils or lotions, or they eat foods rich in vitamin E, C, zinc, and silica and keep their weight gain to the recommended twenty-five pounds during pregnancy. An ounce of prevention is worth a pound of cure. But if, like me, you didn't pay much attention to your weight or to your skin during pregnancy, you're stuck with curing rather than preventing stretch marks.

Studies have shown that prescription creams containing hyaluronic acid (to plump), retinol (to increase collagen), or tretinoin (to resurface and strengthen the skin) reduce the appearance of stretch marks. Over-the-counter creams, such as Mederma and *Cosmopolitan* magazine's number-one choice, Manuela Lubin Delicate Beauty Advanced Stretch Mark Removal Cream (*cosmopolitan.com*, "13 Top Stretch Removal Creams"), appear to work well for some people. The American Association of Dermatology, *aad.org*, has some suggestions for muting the look of stretch marks after delivery. According to the organization, "If you want to try one of these creams, lotions, or gels to fade stretch marks, be sure to:

- Use the product on early stretch marks. Treatment seems to have little effect on mature stretch marks.
- Massage the product into your stretch marks. Taking time to massage the product gently into your skin may make it more effective.
- Apply the product every day for two weeks. If you see results, they take weeks to appear."

A dermatologist may suggest other methods to help reduce stretch marks, such as chemical peels or laser therapies. On the other hand, you may like your souvenirs of pregnancy and choose not to do anything. Again, always get the okay from your medical professional before using creams and potions.

BIGGER FEET

When my feet swelled to a colossal size eleven during the last few weeks of pregnancy, I figured they'd return to their pre-pregnancy size after delivery; after all, most of the swelling was from extra water, right? For years I hung on to my beautiful Guess, size seven-and-a-half, open-toed, "fuck-me" shoes, until I finally realized my feet would never fit into them again. I ended up donating them, along with several other pairs of size seven and eight to my smaller-shoe-sized sister. In the meantime, I would shop the clearance aisles at the discount shoe stores, thinking my feet would eventually shrink back. Today I'm buying shoes that fit well, and I care more about comfort than getting laid! That reminds me of another one of my mother's pearls of wisdom, "Always, always wear a 'good' pair of shoes to prevent problems in the future."

My new size-nine foot can be explained by two things that happen during pregnancy—weight gain and the hormone relaxin. Weight gain can flatten the arch of your foot. Relaxin relaxes the muscle ligaments and alters cartilage and tendons to prepare us for childbirth. Relaxing the pelvis and softening the cervix are the most obvious results of this hormone, but relaxin also eases muscle ligaments in other areas, including the feet. The overall effect can be permanently flattened and lengthened feet.

All I need is a well-fitting pair of shoes to chase my two miracles around the house without breaking an ankle.

LABIA

I haven't put a mirror down there to see for myself, but it's pretty normal for skin color to change down there. It can get darker due to increased blood flow triggered by increased estrogen and progesterone levels during pregnancy. Some women report their labia are longer or that they hang differently after delivery. The inner lips (labia minora) can become so enlarged they rub against clothing, causing irritation, urinary tract infections, and decreased confidence during sexual activity. Quite frankly, they become so prominent in some women, it appears as though they have a small penis or a very hairy bush—especially if they're wearing tight yoga pants or a wet swimsuit (*plasticsurgery.org*).

Sometimes the labia can shrink. The American Association of Plastic Surgery reported 11,218 labiaplasty procedures in 2019, up nine percent from the previous year. Just an FYI, the average cost of the surgery was $2,894 (*plasticsurgery.org / documents/News/Statistics/2019/plastic-surgery-statistics-full-report-2019.pdf.*)

ALL BOOBIES GREAT & SMALL

About a year after having my second baby, I noticed my boobs almost hit the floor when I took off my bra. Okay, I'm exaggerating just a little, but seriously, I felt like Maxine, the cranky old lady from Hallmark greeting cards. The medical name for saggy breasts is "breast ptosis," often referred to as a "rock-in-the-sock" look. My saggy breasts were probably the result of my skin continually expanding to accommodate the sixty-plus pounds I gained during nine months of pregnancy.

After delivery, my breasts became engorged and grew another couple of cup sizes. After that, weaning and a smidge of weight loss caused my breasts to contract. Then I went through it all over again with baby number two. Now, years after my second delivery, one of my nipples points southwest while the other nipple points southeast. They used to stick straight out like a car's headlights, especially on cold days. Now I have to lean back almost into a bridge position to get them to point true north. My once-beautiful Mount Everest breasts now look like a couple of worn-out saddlebags. It's become so difficult to find a bikini that lifts the "girls." No longer can I wear a swimsuit without major underwiring. Try finding a cute bikini with a built-in lift that's not hanging in the women's-plus section or the old-lady aisle. I have to read the small print if I buy one online because the models appear to have had surgical breast lifts, making every bikini top look like a WOW! I've resorted to the tankini and frumpy one-piece section of the store. No longer can I shop the swimsuit aisles for the body I had before children. I guess it's time to suck it up and spend the money on a proper ladies' swimsuit and bra from a specialty shop with help from professional dressers who can outfit my new body shape. Otherwise, I'll be shopping for a swimsuit (or a swimming costume, as we say in jolly old England) in the picked-over clearance section at Target.

The American Society of Plastic Surgeons (ASPS) reported 113,188 breast lift procedures performed by ASPS certified surgeons in 2019, compared to 109,638 breast lift surgeries in 2018—up three percent year to year (*plasticsurgery.org/ documents/News/Statistics/2019*). Breast lift procedures have grown by 114 percent since the year 2000. Although breast implant surgeries are the most commonly performed cosmetic surgery in women, with 299,715 procedures in 2019, breast lift surgeries are catching up. Women aged thirty to fifty-four made up almost seventy percent of mastopexy (breast lift) surgeries in 2019. *Allure* magazine nailed the reason why (*allure.com/story/types-ofbreast-lift-surgery by Joan Kron*):

"After decades of wanting bigger, round breasts, women are increasingly choosing altitude over amplitude...This suggests that the newest trend in breast surgery isn't the quest for what you've never had, but instead for what you've lost."

Quite a few of my mommy friends compare themselves to "Sisters, Not Twins." I was intrigued, so, of course, I googled "uneven boobs" and came across a great article published in *SELF*, November 2017, written by Korin Miller. She interviewed a doctor who said it's actually more common for women to have different-shaped breasts than symmetrical breasts. Blame genetics. Another article I enjoyed reading was from *thehealthy.com/breast-health/uneven-breasts/*, which talks about changing breast shapes after pregnancy. Blame hormones. FYI, most of my friends report their left boob being bigger than their right boob. Fact or fiction?

ALL BOOBIES GREAT and SMALL

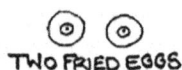

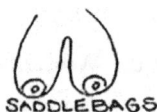

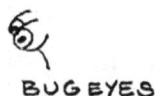

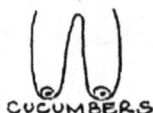

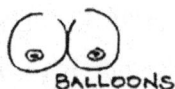

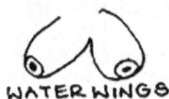

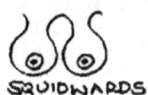

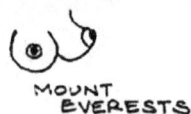

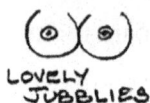

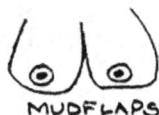

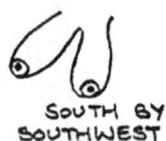

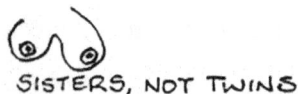

TWO FRIED EGGS

SADDLEBAGS

BUG EYES

CUCUMBERS

BUG BITES

BALLOONS

WATER WINGS

SQUIDWARDS

MOUNT EVERESTS

LOVELY JUBBLIES

MUDFLAPS

SOUTH BY SOUTHWEST

SISTERS, NOT TWINS

CHAPTER 16

TOOT-TOOT, TRAIN COMING

Growing up, my three brothers thought the funniest thing in the world was to trap me in a Dutch Oven. I'd retaliate with my super stealthy, "silent but deadly" arsenal of gas-antics. After my episiotomy, I lost my duplicitous ability. Now, especially after a couple of beers, I can clear a room in seconds with my thunderous farts.

The *Daily Mail* online newspaper published a story in 2014 about an opera singer who sued the US government because a nurse at an army hospital in Kentucky gave her an episiotomy that left her soiling herself and farting like a trombone. The piece was headlined, "Opera Singer, 33, 'suffered botched episiotomy that led to excessive flatulence and left her unable to perform.'"

At first glance, the headline appears a little humorous and far-fetched, but I'm living proof that bowel health can change after childbirth. My "lack of control of my flatus" and my occasional "bowel urgency" are two symptoms associated with anal incontinence (although, on second thought, my bowel urgency may be the result of a good curry or a very spicy taco).

Most women suffer from a bit of gas or stool leakage after delivery, especially with vaginal delivery; it's normal. The "Subway Sandwich" is adept at catching any leakage and muffling the sound of gas so most women don't even notice. It usually resolves within a few weeks. If, however, you had an episiotomy or an assisted delivery with forceps, you might be plagued with embarrassing escapes for years after having children. *Aboutincontinence.org* and MASIC (Mothers with Anal Injuries in Childbirth) list nerve damage from the baby's head moving through the birth canal, damage to the pelvic floor muscles from forceps, and tears to the anal sphincter as three probable causes for flatulence and poop problems down the road.

The website *www.aboutincontinence.org* describes anal incontinence, or bowel incontinence (and I quote):

"Bowel urgency means that there is very little time (five minutes or less) between the first urge to have a bowel movement and the need to pass stool. Bowel incontinence includes involuntary leakage or loss of control of gas, liquid stool, mucous, or solid stool. Bowel urgency and incontinence to gas are particularly common in the first few months after vaginal delivery. (Urinary urgency and incontinence are also very common during this time.)"

Nursingtimes.net has a great explanation of the subject. The website reports that five percent of all women giving birth annually in the United Kingdom sustain an injury to the anal sphincter during vaginal delivery. The website says that upon later reexamination of these women, the actual number of injuries could be as high as eleven to 24.5 percent (Andrews et al. 2006). Unfortunately, many women fail to seek treatment because they don't recognize that they sustained an injury, and, in addition, they're overwhelmed with shame and embarrassment. A more recent study cited by *webmd.com/baby/news*, "Incontinence After Childbirth May Last Years," suggests that two percent of births in the United States each year leave women with persistent long-term anal incontinence. The May 2020 article also states that only about ten percent of these women report their symptoms to their healthcare providers. The condition can negatively impact a woman's quality of life and a mother's ability to care for and bond with her child.

I would never have put two and two together. I noticed my flatulence increase after I had my first baby. I figured everything changes after childbirth, so my augmented habit of "floating an air biscuit" was just another oddity to add to the list. My gas problem became more of an issue a few years after my second baby was born. I blamed the dog for my loud bottom burps that crept out at the most inopportune times. It came to the point where I finally plucked up the nerve to mention my flatulence to my family doctor. She suggested I try the low FODMAP diet (reducing the number of foods high in Fermentables, Oligosaccharides, Disaccharides, Monosaccharides, and Polyols). She handed me a list of foods on the high short-chain carbohydrate and sugar alcohol side and told me to avoid them. Trying to follow her direction, I limited garlic, onions, dairy, gluten, and grains, but I had so little left in the pantry to work with for someone who enjoys cooking. I have to say, by cutting out the high FODMAP foods, my gas subsided. However, after researching more about anal incontinence, I returned to my tasty staples and subsequently blamed my gas on childbirth; I find it hard to live without garlic, onions, mushrooms, apples, avocado, milk, and pasta. Who's going to argue with me for cutting the cheese if I explain I have a small pelvic opening that led to an emergency episiotomy during delivery—I may have an injured sphincter?!

FYI, *IBSDiets.org* has a list of foods you can and can't eat if you want to give the low FODMAP diet a go.

CHAPTER 17:

WHERE DID I LEAVE MY MIND? (THE MEMORY LOSS CONTINUES)

While you were pregnant, did you find yourself forgetting certain words and asking people to pass, "that thing"? Were you continually drawing a blank on the names of items when the item is sitting right in front of you? You know, that "thing" that holds water, sitting in the middle of the lunch table? I'm thirsty and need a refill.

Did you have similar experiences, like walking into a room and forgetting why you're there? Going to the store and forgetting what you need? Driving through McDonald's, paying at the first window, then driving off without stopping at the second window to collect your food? I'm sure it was just as frustrating for people to be around us as it was for us to go through this phase of pregnancy forgetfulness.

You may think all will return to normal after the baby is born. Not so fast. I still feel like a vacationer abroad, unable to speak the native language fluently. No doubt you'll be watching a slew of kids' movies as your little one grows. One of our family favorites is *The Incredibles*. In the second movie, Mr. Incredible, Bob, takes care of his three children while Elastigirl, his wife, goes back to work to save the city. Their youngest child is a baby, their second child is ten, and their oldest is a teenager. Bob becomes so exhausted from becoming the primary caregiver, he laments, "I haven't been sleeping. I broke my daughter; they keep changing math; we need AA batteries, but I got AAAs, and now we still need AA batteries. I put one red thing in a load of whites, and now everything's pink. I think we need eggs." I completely feel his pain.

Can we blame this side effect of parenthood on fluctuating hormone levels, too? Or is it more to do with sleep deprivation, a lifestyle shift, or something else? Is "mommy brain" a real thing?

In my experience, my baby always came first, so who cares if I forgot the word "pitcher"? I didn't need to know the name of particular objects to care for my baby. It was almost like I became a mothering machine, programmed to, first and foremost, tend to my baby. I became so adept at figuring out the meaning of her cries, from her tired cry, wet diaper cry, her hungry, "feed me now!" cry. My body was programmed to cultivate her every need. My breasts leaked when my baby needed feeding. After my baby woke from a nap, I knew I had to check her diaper. My sleep pattern mirrored my baby's sleep pattern. For the first few weeks, my body wasn't my own; it positively responded to my baby's needs, which was okay, because my baby and I were both new to this. As the months went by, I started remembering the names of objects again. I became more in control of my body, and my baby became less and less dependent on me.

The New York Times published an article in May 2018 called "Reframing Mommy Brain." It states that during pregnancy, and for some time after delivery, we may forget someone's name, but our ability to learn, reason, and comprehend is not affected. The article says there's no real evidence to suggest pregnancy causes a decline in mental processing or memory; instead, our brain can shift focus in response to new experiences. We may forget to pick up dry cleaning, for instance, in exchange for growth in emotional processing in response to having a baby. In essence, "mommy brain" may make us more forgetful of the trivial, but our ability to understand is not affected. Forgetting things may make us good parents. We change to become responsive to our babies' needs. We're not losing our smarts; we're merely rearranging our brain's strengths to better bond with and care for our children.

Interestingly, "mommy brain" isn't exclusive to women. A study published in the journal *Proceedings of the National*

Academy of Sciences in 2014 by Abraham et al. (*pnas.org*) used MRI imagery to study activity patterns of the brain in first-time parents. There were three groups of parents:

1. Heterosexual moms who were primary caregivers to their infant
2. Heterosexual dads who were secondary caregivers to their infant
3. Homosexual dads who were primary caregivers to their infant and had no maternal involvement

The authors of the study looked at how the brain changes in response to stimuli from their babies. In addition to MRI, they looked at oxytocin levels and parenting behavior. Brain patterns changed as a result of caregiving behavior. Mothers and primary-caregiving fathers exhibited high activation of the amygdala compared to secondary caregivers. The amygdala is an almond-shaped part of the brain located in the middle temporal lobe; part of the limbic system, it's responsible for emotional processing. According to *Britannica*, it's known to be involved in positive emotions elicited by rewarding stimuli. So, regardless of being male or female, if we're primary caregivers actively engaged in caring for our infant, our brain is stimulated similarly.

I don't think everything goes back to normal entirely, however. I'm not sure if I can use the excuse, but I continue to experience "mommy brain" many years after delivery. My child is still dependent on me eleven years later, but her dependency isn't for breastfeeding or a diaper change; it's for love, guidance, and emotional support. I still forget the names of words, albeit to a lesser extent. As for my overall forgetfulness, I currently make lists to help me remember. If I don't write milk or eggs on the grocery list right away, my fridge will be bare, or chores don't get done. I predict I will continue to ask someone to pass that "thing" for as long as I'm a mom. After all, a mother's work "is never done," right?

CHAPTER 18

WHEN IS THE BABY DUE?

No, I'm not pregnant! I may look like I am, but trust me, I'm not; after all, "It's Shark Week!" That line should nip the quizzing in the bud. "Are you sure you're not pregnant?" People think they have a sixth sense, confident they know someone's pregnant when they have no clue. As if I want to go through that all over again. The memories are still so vivid. And yes, two years after delivery, I still had a soft, squidgy, giant belly pooch. I couldn't imagine adding more poundage to a body that screams, "I'm the next contender for the *Biggest Loser* TV show."

Eleven years postpartum, I'm nowhere near my pre-pregnancy size six. Granted, I put on sixty pounds during my first pregnancy. Okay, sixty-six pounds—like Kate Hudson during one of her pregnancies. I convinced myself I was eating for two, and therefore I could eat anything I wanted anytime, anyplace, anywhere. But unlike Kate Hudson, who quickly lost her pregnancy weight, I kept telling myself, "I'll start my diet tomorrow." Growing up, my mother had a slew of expressions in response to my procrastination, such as, "Tomorrow Never Comes," "One Day or Day One?" and my favorite (which I never understood until recently), "Can't Is the Won't, for People Who Don't." Thanks, Mom; I know now.

Let's not compare ourselves to movie stars. Kate Hudson had a movie role waiting for her that paid her big bucks. She was motivated to lose weight quickly. If I had a million-dollar carrot dangling in front of me, I'd be more proactive, too. Realistically, though, to help her lose her additional pounds, she ate high-protein meals in small quantities and exercised. Her workout programs included cardiovascular exercise and weight training (just like the *Biggest Loser!*). She had a "normal" post-pregnancy body after giving birth, but not a Hollywood post-pregnancy body, which is entirely unrealistic. She received so much flak for the extra weight she'd gained that she set her goal high and lost the baby weight in just four months. She also regained abdominal muscles that were Hollywood's envy and soon looked smoking hot in a bikini. The lesson here is losing weight quickly is doable. We all know we should eat healthily and work out, it's no secret, but **it isn't easy!** In an interview with *People* magazine, Kate Hudson's advice was to stick to the basics and be disciplined. But then again, many movie stars can afford to pay for top personal trainers and nutritionists, unlike me. They can also afford to pay for babysitters or nannies to take care of children while they work out. Until I had a baby, I didn't realize the value of a good babysitter. I didn't have a network of sitters waiting in the wings. I would beg, borrow, or steal for free time, just to sleep. I give Kate enormous kudos for her discipline and commitment. My mind wasn't in the same place.

Unfortunately, there's a lot of unrealistic pressure on women to look a certain way, even after having a baby. Photographs of svelte Hollywood stars morphing into heavy versions of themselves always make the front pages of popular magazines. We're secretly comforted to know stars are human, just like us. Callie Ahlgrim wrote an uplifting article published in *Insider.com* in April 2019 titled, "24 times celebrity moms were refreshingly honest about their post-pregnancy bodies." A-list personalities spoke candidly about their bigger butts, thighs, and waists after having their babies. Many of these ladies reiterated that there's nothing natural about losing baby weight quickly, and they celebrated their soft tummies and new size. Jennifer Garner actually named her post-baby tummy bump Violet, Sam, and Sera (her three children's names) because false pregnancy rumors swirled after she had her third child.

After having her second child in 2016, Pink wrote in an Instagram message, "Would you believe I'm 160lbs and 5′3″?

By regular standards, that makes me obese. I know I'm not at my goal or anywhere near it after baby two, but dammit, I don't feel obese. The only thing I'm feeling is myself. Stay off that scale ladies!"

As they say, nine months on, nine months off. When my daughter was nine months old, I was shopping for my clothes at the secondhand thrift store. I kept thinking I'd start losing weight tomorrow, so I didn't want to invest in expensive clothing—and the thrift stores around me are excellent. I bought a whole new wardrobe for around a hundred bucks, including brand-name clothes from the Banana Republic, Façonnable, The Gap, St. John (oh yeah baby, seventeen dollars for a mint-condition St. John jacket), Tommy Bahama, and Reebok. I refused to spend a lot of money on clothes during my postpartum weight-loss period. I took three months of maternity leave after having my baby, and it took me a while to adjust to going back to work full time. The last thing on my mind was working to lose the baby weight. And, at the end of the workday, I couldn't wait to pick up my little one from daycare. Her excitement to see me walk through the door was priceless.

Losing weight does get easier as time goes by. My priorities changed after having a baby, and losing weight wasn't my number-one goal for quite some time. For the first few years,

I was okay with my new "Mom" body. Sure, it stings a little when you walk into a bar and heads don't turn anymore, but I'm proud of what I created and wouldn't change my situation for the world. I wasn't in a rush to return to my pre-pregnancy size six. Like everything in life, it's about mentally preparing yourself and continually praising and rewarding yourself for every inch of progress made. A glance in the mirror and a look that says, "Oh yeah, Baby! You've got this!"

FYI, daycare is an excellent place to find a babysitter! Sidebar, some more of my favorite expressions from my mother include, "If a Job's Worth Doing, It's Worth Doing Well." "Don't be a Half-a-Job Harry," "A Stitch in Time Saves Nine," "Know Your Onions," "Stir with a Knife, Stir up Strife," and, "Don't Trip over the Pounds (Dollars) to Pick up the Pennies."

CHAPTER 19

SWEATY CROTCH

After bladder sling surgery, I welcomed the idea of exercising again. I started to play tennis, which is a sport I wouldn't have dreamed of playing before the fix—running all over the court, back and forth, side to side, sprinting, reaching, stretching, twisting, and jumping. I hadn't exerted myself for more than seven years, not since mid-pregnancy with my first. No wonder I was carrying so much extra "baby" weight. Now I had the freedom to move quickly and suddenly without embarrassing bladder squirts.

Why then, after my workouts on the tennis court, did I end a session with a wet gusset? It didn't make sense; I'd had the fix! I wasn't peeing myself anymore. The soggy triangle in the front of my shorts, I discovered, was the result of crotch sweat. Even during my days of running 5Ks, I never ended a race with a sweaty crotch, but now, postpartum, after exerting myself, I end up with a swamp crotch.

Vaginas don't have sweat glands, so it wasn't coming from there. We have a bunch of sweat glands in the pelvic and groin areas. Our hairy parts have apocrine glands that release a thick sweat, thicker than sweat from other parts of our body. Pubic hair can trap sweat and make it hard for it to escape. But the whole point of sweating is to cool our skin—as the water in sweat evaporates, the surface of the skin cools. And that's true of sweat from eccrine glands. It's thinner and evaporates quickly to cool down the temperature of the skin. Apocrine is different; it's the stinky kind of a sweat. If it hangs around too long and mixes with bacteria, it can smell rancid.

Self.com magazine, in an article published online in April 2019 by Korin Miller, explains that doctors don't know why we produce apocrine sweat. Many animals in the animal kingdom produce it. It gives off pheromones to attract other animals. I'm not sure what my husband thinks of my sweaty crotch after three sets of tennis, but I've had enough of it! I took to the internet. Wearing tight workout pants can help trap apocrine sweat. Wearing pads or panty liners can also act as traps. Carrying extra body weight, especially around the thighs and the hip areas, can produce friction while exercising and therefore produce more heat in the groin area. Finally, having a hairy groin can trap the dreaded apocrine sweat.

I'm heavier than I used to be and I'm pear-shaped, so I carry more weight down below. Running around the tennis court produces a lot of friction! I don't shave or trim as often as I used to before having children—usually only before date night or an OB appointment, because time alone in the shower takes planning these days. But now I know what I can do to help alleviate sweaty crotch—trim, shave, wear loose-fitting, breathable clothing (waiting for my TommyJohn bra and panties to arrive) and keep working out to help lose weight. Got it!

CHAPTER 20

THE MOMMY MAKEOVER

A friend of mine told me she would start saving her money for a tummy tuck after she completed her family. How extravagant and completely unnecessary, I thought. She didn't look overweight. In fact, she looked great. I always admired her killer legs in a short dress. Her body is an apple shape. She told me that after her first pregnancy, she ended up with folds of extra skin around her belly that hung like the soft wrinkles of a tired, deflated balloon.

During my first pregnancy, I looked like a tick so full it could burst at any minute. I ballooned to an all-time high of 212 pounds during pregnancy. My skin was stretched so tight. I only lost a total of twenty-six pounds after my delivery and months later, I still sported a soft, squidgy tummy with noticeable excess skin. I'd heard some friends talk about a "Mommy Makeover" and wanted to know more. They talked about either a full or a partial makeover. I couldn't quite picture what was involved, so I took to the internet and googled it. Holy Momma! I found photos of women's torsos before and after the makeovers. The differences were striking. I learned that a full makeover includes a breast lift, liposuction around the flank, and abdominoplasty, also known as a tummy tuck. The partial makeover is an a la carte version of the full.

Abdominoplasty involves the repair of separated connective tissue between the abdominal muscles. A surgeon goes in and sews the muscles or tissue back together and removes any excess skin and fat from the middle and lower abdomen. Apparently, no matter how hard we crunch, if our muscles are separated more than two finger spaces, our killer six-pack stomach isn't happening without a little intervention. DRAM, diastasis of the rectus abdomens muscle, or diastasis (separation) recti, occurs when the two long, parallel, rectus abdominis muscles that run vertically from our chest to our pelvis get stretched from our growing uterus during pregnancy. The connective tissue between the muscles, called linea alba, acts like a stretchy rubber band. Sometimes this tissue stretches too much and has a hard time bouncing back, leaving a gap between the muscles, which makes us look like we're still pregnant months later. Ever noticed how women having their first baby often don't show for a few months, but women pregnant with their second, third, or fifth baby seem to pop much earlier? Stretched connective tissue is probably the culprit. [4]

During the first eight weeks after delivery, many women recover from separated connective tissue, and then recovery plateaus after that. According to the Cleveland Clinic, sixty percent of women are affected during pregnancy and during the postpartum recovery period, and forty percent of those women are still affected six months after delivery. With very little muscle around the belly button to hold in the tummy, organs, and overlying tissue, some women end up with a bulge. The bulge can be an organ poking through, also known as a hernia. Herniated organs are not only painful but can be dangerous. Back pain can also be a painful side effect of diastasis recti. There are exercises to help put the connective tissue back in place, or a surgical option is a tummy tuck. Be sure to consult your physician before starting any exercises, especially if you suspect separated tummy muscles, because not all abdominal exercises will help.

After stretching out a second time with baby number two, I seriously considered a tummy tuck. I wrestled with a number of thoughts. How painful would the surgery be? Would I be able to sit up in bed without using my arms to push myself

---

4   The UK's National Health Service has a website that gives instructions on how to measure the gap between your muscles. Check out *www.nhs.uk your-post-pregnancy-body.*

into position? How much would it cost? Am I being too vain for wanting to lose my marks of motherhood, namely, my muffin tops, loose belly skin, my squidgy tummy, and maybe even a few stretch marks?

My daughter's school, like many schools, holds an auction every year to raise money to pay for additional teacher development programs and education. I bought a gift certificate for eyelash extensions donated by a plastic surgery office in town. I very quickly fell in love with eyelash extensions—who has time for mascara in the morning with two kids to get ready? I soon discovered the office staff was very professional, and so I started to ask my friends if they knew anything about the skills of the plastic surgeons who practiced there. It was surprising how many women came out of the woodwork to tell me the procedures they'd had done at the very same clinic. One friend had had a breast reduction, another a breast lift, another friend had a tummy tuck, and another had liposuction performed around her thighs, bra fat, and midsection. No wonder my friends looked so good!

My esthetician recommended a couple of board-certified plastic surgeons to consult, and the consultation was free. The American Society of Plastic Surgeons (ASPS) lists a number of questions on its website you may want to ask your surgeon during a consult. Some important questions include, is your surgeon board-certified? How many years have they been practicing plastic surgery? Do they have hospital privileges? What does the recovery look like? Am I a good candidate for plastic surgery, or would I be a better candidate for a laser treatment such as CoolSculpting that freezes and eliminates fat cells? The ASPS also has a list of the most common causes of a loose, sagging, or protruding abdomen, and those factors include aging, heredity, pregnancy, prior surgery, and significant fluctuations in weight. I'd established I could check four of the five main causes: age, C-section surgery, and significant weight gain (and not so much the loss) from pregnancy.

I decided it was time to make an appointment to talk to a surgeon.

I must admit, I was nervous as I sat in the patient room waiting for my doctor to enter. All kinds of thoughts were whizzing through my head. Why can't I lose weight myself, the old-fashioned way, with diet and exercise? Am I being vain and insecure in resorting to surgery? How much would it cost? Can I afford a mommy makeover? By the end of the consult, I decided to spend my money on a good bra rather than a breast lift; however, I did schedule surgery for abdominoplasty/tummy tuck. My surgeon confirmed that during pregnancy, it's common for the abdominal muscles to weaken and separate. In my head, I heard, "So with diet and exercise, it's almost impossible to lose my sagging skin and retrieve my tight, flat tummy as I had before pregnancy." He told me I'd be a good candidate for the surgery and that I'd be wearing a bikini by the time he was finished with me. Really? This body hadn't seen a bikini in years, not since before pregnancy. I'd thrown out most of my bikinis long ago. I doubted his words and told him I'd be wearing tankinis and a coverup forever. But I was wrong.

Only six weeks post-surgery, I was wearing a slinky black-and-white two-piece. Not a tankini, but a bikini that showed off most of my midsection. My surgeon had removed excess fat from around my flank, my back, and my tummy. Although a tummy tuck isn't considered a weight-loss tool, I'd lost eighteen pounds and my stomach was flat and tight. I could see a six-pack emerging and I felt great. My love handles had disappeared, and I felt confident wearing shapely sports tops, which in turn made me want to exercise more.

This procedure is considered major surgery, and the recovery was lengthy—about five to six weeks. The first week was by far the hardest because I was bedridden for the most part. My surgeon had injected a liquid prior to the liposuction, a mixture of saline solution, lidocaine, and epinephrine. After surgery, the liquid leaked out of the incisions he'd made to suck out the fat. It was bright red and looked like Kool-Aid. I laid a fifty-gallon trash bag on top of my mattress, topped it with a couple of beach towels, and a sizeable hospital incontinence absorbent bed pad. I leaked for about two or three days, and my torso was bruised and swollen. My doctor gave me an elasticated compression band that I wore day and night to help control the swelling.

The incision from my tummy tuck ran across the entire front of my body, beginning just beyond my left hip bone, curving down to my pubic hair, and curving back up, ending just beyond my right hip bone. Measuring a whopping nineteen inches long, the incision was very painful, especially when I moved. I had to roll out of bed for bathroom visits. I had two drainage tubes, one sticking out of each end of the incision. The tubes emptied into bags that slowly collected a bloody liquid. My doctor instructed me to empty the bags a few times a day and measure the amount of fluid my body was discharging. It was pretty scary at first, but I soon got the hang of it. After a week, I returned to my doctor's office for the removal of the tubes, after which, I felt much more mobile and a lot less fragile.

My belly button is mine, but the original skin all around it was cut away during surgery. The remaining skin was pulled down and sewn together. A new hole was made through which my belly button now appears. At first, my belly button looked like a tiny sun with rays of small scars all the way around it. I have an "inny." Years later, the scars are hardly noticeable.

My children were three years and eight years old at the time of my surgery, so they were somewhat self-sufficient with the help of Daddy. My doctor loaded me up with prescriptions to help me through the first week. Armed with Valium to help prevent muscle spasms, Oxycodone to ease the pain, and the support of my loving husband, it almost felt as though I was on vacation. I caught up on movies, and my own Netflix shows (no Disney or Nickelodeon). I was waited on hand and foot as I lay in bed all day. Once again, I felt like Kristin Bell in the movie *Bad Moms* as she sits at a bar telling her fellow "Bad Moms" Mila Kunis and Kathryn Hahn, "Sometimes when I'm driving all by myself, I have this fantasy that I get into a car crash. Not a big one with fire and explosions, but just a little one. But I do get injured, and I get to go to the hospital for two weeks, and I sleep all day and I eat Jell-O and watch TV, and it's all covered by my insurance." Having alone time while recovering from surgery was kind of like that, only mine wasn't covered by insurance!

The doctor's orders included no lifting any more than ten pounds for the first couple of weeks, and no lifting more than twenty-five pounds for an additional four weeks after that. I have amazing friends who came to my house and washed and folded laundry for me. I'd stocked the fridge and freezer with prepared meals ahead of my procedure, so all my husband had to do was pop the food in the oven and dinner was ready. I'd also planned the surgery during summer vacation. That way we could all relax for the first week. I'm lucky my oldest child enjoys snuggling with Mommy, so I received plenty of hugs and had a dedicated little helper.

Today, the incision scar is hardly noticeable, and bikini bottoms and panties cover it completely. My stomach is flat, and the best part is that my core is strong. I can sit up using only my abdominal muscles, and I can see muscle definition for the first time in years. Would I do it all over again? The answer is yes, it worked for me. I'm lucky I had no complications. Abdominoplasty is definitely a major surgery, so keep that in mind if you decide to have a tummy tuck.

CHAPTER 21:

AND THE DADS WEIGH IN

Daddy, after reading all this, what are your thoughts?

All will be revealed in the next book. Stay tuned!